Praise for *The Ethical Lives of Clients: Transcending Self-Interest in Psychotherapy*

Clinicians rarely have the opportunity to examine their own ethical and moral stances in light of challenging client questions. Bill Doherty expertly provides a clear path to examine issues from a relational perspective, and sheds light on critical issues for mental health professionals at all levels.
—**Terence Patterson, EdD, ABPP,** Board Certified Couple and Family Psychologist; Fellow, American Psychological Association; and coauthor of *Real-World Couple Counseling and Therapy*

Doherty's book is a logical extension of his previous groundbreaking work on relational ethics in therapy and provides the "something more" we all need to practice ethically sensitive therapy ourselves.
—**Fred P. Piercy, PhD,** Professor Emeritus, College of Liberal Arts and Human Sciences, Virginia Tech, Blacksburg, VA, and Former Editor, *Journal of Marital and Family Therapy*

The Ethical Lives of Clients is one of the most important books to appear about psychotherapy in a generation. Dr. Doherty brings the sorts of ethical choices clients and therapists face clearly into focus, moving us out of the frame of the technical aspects of what to do in psychotherapy to the moral aspects of our work.
—**Jay Lebow, PhD, ABPP,** The Family Institute at Northwestern and Northwestern University, Evanston, IL, and Editor, *Family Process*

THE
ETHICAL
LIVES OF
CLIENTS

THE ETHICAL LIVES OF CLIENTS

Transcending Self-Interest in Psychotherapy

WILLIAM J. DOHERTY

 AMERICAN PSYCHOLOGICAL ASSOCIATION

Published by
American Psychological Association
750 First Street, NE
Washington, DC 20002
https://www.apa.org

Order Department
https://www.apa.org/pubs/books
order@apa.org

In the U.K., Europe, Africa, and the Middle East, copies may be ordered from Eurospan
https://www.eurospanbookstore.com/apa
info@eurospangroup.com

Typeset in Charter and Interstate by Circle Graphics, Inc., Reisterstown, MD

Printer: Sheridan Books, Chelsea, MI
Cover Designer: Gwen J. Grafft, Minneapolis, MN

Library of Congress Cataloging-in-Publication Data

Names: Doherty, William J. (William Joseph), 1945- author.
Title: The ethical lives of clients : transcending self-interest in
  psychotherapy / William J. Doherty.
Description: Washington, DC : American Psychological Association, [2022] |
  Includes bibliographical references and index.
Identifiers: LCCN 2021019713 (print) | LCCN 2021019714 (ebook) |
  ISBN 9781433836565 (paperback) | ISBN 9781433837463 (ebook)
Subjects: LCSH: Ethical therapy. | Self-interest. | Psychotherapist and patient.
Classification: LCC RC489.E83 D64 2022 (print) | LCC RC489.E83 (ebook) |
  DDC 616.89/14—dc23
LC record available at https://lccn.loc.gov/2021019713
LC ebook record available at https://lccn.loc.gov/2021019714

https://doi.org/10.1037/0000263-000

Printed in the United States of America

10 9 8 7 6 5 4 3 2

Contents

THE
ETHICAL
LIVES OF
CLIENTS

INTRODUCTION

The Ethical Domain of Clients' Lives

Laura is a middle-aged woman with two teenagers and a difficult mother who is long widowed, in her late 70s, and living in another state.[1] Her mother calls Laura regularly to complain about her life (her one good friend has recently died) and her increasing ailments. She criticizes Laura for how she is handling her own life, including her mothering. Laura dreads these long calls, feels guilty as an only child for not supporting her mother more, and recoils from her mother's criticisms. Increasingly torn about how to manage her mother, her self-care, and her other life responsibilities, Laura called me for therapy.

This is a garden-variety psychotherapy scenario with plenty to explore in terms of the history of the mother–daughter relationship, Laura's difficulty in setting boundaries, and other issues. Here's an additional complication: Laura is getting advice from her friends to simply cut off her relationship with her mother—"drop her," in the words of one of her friends, who happens to be a therapist. That feels wrong to Laura, but she wonders whether

---

[1]The case examples in this chapter and throughout the book have been modified to disguise the identities of the clients involved and to protect their confidentiality.

https://doi.org/10.1037/0000263-001

The Ethical Lives of Clients: Transcending Self-Interest in Psychotherapy, by W. J. Doherty

that's because she has become codependent with her mother (an idea she got from a self-help book).

As noted, there is plenty of strictly clinical material to work with here, and in the first half of my career as a therapist, that's all I would have considered. Then I came to realize that clients like Laura have an ethical dilemma wrapped up in their personal challenges. In this case, it was about her obligations as the only offspring of an increasingly frail mother. Like many other ethical dilemmas, this one took the form of a tension between needs of self—for Laura, reduced stress and burden—and responsibilities to other people in our lives.

Later in this book, I describe how I work with clients such as Laura. For now, I want to clarify that this book is about the ethics of clients and how we work with their ethical dilemmas and not about ethical issues for therapists. There is a vast literature on professional ethical issues such as respecting client autonomy, maintaining confidentiality, and so forth (e.g., Knapp et al., 2017; Wilcoxon et al., 2011). But there is relatively little guidance for therapists on how to help clients facing their own ethical dilemmas such as to divorce or remain in a miserable marriage, to continue a secret affair or end it, to cut off or stay connected with a difficult family member, to lie or be truthful when the truth might create conflict, to keep a family secret or tell others—the list is long. And then there are ethical issues that the client may not see but the therapist does, such as a divorced parent undermining the child's relationship with a despised ex-spouse, or a client with a sexually transmitted disease who does not feel a need to inform sexual partners. Cutting across these examples is a core element of human life: the tension between personal needs and desires on the one hand and the potential harm we can cause others as we act on those needs and desires on the other.

For the purposes of this book, I use the terms *ethical* and *moral* interchangeably and define them as decisions and actions that have consequences for the welfare of others. My rationale for using these terms interchangeably is pragmatic. From presenting ideas in this book over the years, I have learned that when the term *moral* is used on its own, many therapists hear it as connoting negative judgment—it sounds like "moralistic." Therapists seem not to have the same wary response to the term *ethical*, which is commonly used in the field for therapists' own behavior and which I am relating to the world of clients. However, I do not want to abandon the term *moral* altogether, and in fact, I review literature from the field of moral psychology. Hence, the decision to use both terms. On the definition of the moral domain as involving decisions and actions that have consequences for the welfare of others, I am again being pragmatic. There is a long tradition of debate among philosophers about what constitutes the domain of ethics (e.g., Crisp, 2015). For reasons more fully described in Chapter 6, I come down on a practical, relational definition that focuses on clients' choices and behaviors that have a meaningful impact on the well-being of people in their lives, in particular, avoiding harming others. Ethics here deals with accountability for how we treat others.

The principal argument of this book is that because we humans are ethical creatures who regularly deal with issues of right and wrong, of self-interest and responsibility to others, psychotherapy is truncated if it ignores the ethical dimension of our clients' lives. There is no separating psychological well-being from the client's sense of ethical integrity. In this light, I believe we have overlooked the ethical dimension in the lives of people who come to psychotherapy and that this neglect stems from an overly individualistic view of the human person, a view that dominates Western consumer culture. At a broad conceptual level, I propose an expanded view of the relational self, which inevitably involves responsibilities and commitments as part of the core of identity. I use moral foundations theory (Haidt & Joseph, 2007) to identify moral emotions that clients (and all of us) bring to their ethical decisions and dilemmas. On the ground level, as therapists interact with clients dealing with moral concerns, I offer many case examples of a set of skills using the acronym LEAP-C (listen, explore, affirm, perspective—challenge).

HISTORICAL NEGLECT OF THE ETHICAL DOMAIN IN THERAPY

Despite the importance of ethical issues and dilemmas in our clients' lives and their presence in many problems clients bring to therapists, the psychotherapy literature has been nearly silent on this topic. Why do we lack explicit concepts and clinical tools for therapists to use when helping clients with ethical concerns? Partly, I believe, it's because we worry about invading clients' autonomy—pushing our own agenda—if we venture too far into ethics-oriented conversations. I recall a seasoned therapist who treated a lonely, older man whose wife was in a nursing home with advanced Alzheimer's disease. The client was considering dating another woman but agonized about betraying his wife and his marriage vows. After listening and empathizing with the man, the therapist responded, "I'm a therapist, not a priest. Why don't you talk to your priest about this?" Years later, the therapist still did not feel good about his response, but he could not see an alternative approach. As we unpacked the story, he realized that he thought he needed to be an ethical expert to help his client. Because he was not an ethicist and believed that prescribing the client's decision would be contrary to ethical therapy practice, he felt paralyzed and turfed the client to a priest.

At a larger level than therapist discomfort, the neglect of the ethical side of human life is rooted in the historical origins of our field. Freud (1961), the founder of talk therapy, placed morality in the superego, not the ego, and thus outside of the focus of psychoanalytic treatment. The sociologist Phillip Rieff offered a powerful analysis of this issue in two important books published in the mid-20th century: *Freud: The Mind of the Moralist* (1961) and *The Triumph of the Therapeutic: Uses of Faith After Freud* (1966). Rieff (1966) articulated four "character ideals" that have dominated eras of Western history: the political person of classic antiquity, the religious person in Judaism and Christianity until the Enlightenment, the economic person (the Enlightenment through the early 20th century), and then the psychological person whose goal is self-satisfaction and personal insight. "Beginning with Freud," according to Rieff (1966), "the best spirits of the 20th century have thus expressed their conviction that . . . the new center, which can be held even as communities disintegrate, is the self" (p. 10). For Rieff, if the moral realm is reduced to the self, which is the domain of psychology, therapists become de facto moral teachers who focus only on navigating the interests of the self. In other words, the ethical realm disappeared into the clinical realm. Similar critiques have been offered by social scientists and social critics such as Robert Bellah et al. (1985), Christopher Lasch (1979), Michael Lerner (1991), and Michael and Lise Wallach (1983).

This idea of the unfettered, self-made person made its way into mainstream culture by the 1970s, as reflected in the words of the popular writer Gail Sheehy (1976) when she wrote about "the mid-life journey" in her best-selling book *Passages: Predictable Crisis of Adult Life*:

> You can't take everything with you when you leave on the midlife journey. You are moving away. Away from institutional claims and other people's agenda. Away from external valuations and accreditations, in search of an inner validation. You are moving out of roles and into the self. If I could give everyone a gift for the send-off on this journey, it would be a tent. A tent for tentativeness. The gift of portable roots. . . . For each of us there is the opportunity to emerge reborn, authentically unique, with an enlarged capacity to love ourselves and embrace others. . . . The delights of self-discovery are always available. Though loved ones move in and out of our lives, the capacity to love remains. (pp. 364, 513)

On a personal note, I was inspired by words like Sheehy's when I read them at the time. I was in graduate school, and many of us were breaking away from what felt like rigid cultural constraints. But after I witnessed the fruits of so many disposable relationships, I became sobered by the one-sidedness of an emphasis on personal freedom without personal commitments. I came to know Gail Sheehy in the years before her death in 2020 and collaborated with her on a project to promote a broad social good. I never asked her about what she wrote in the mid-1970s, but I would not be surprised if she had tempered her enthusiasm for the gift of tentativeness. We are all products of the collective stories we tell ourselves at different moments in history.

Back to the therapy world: Around the same time as Rieff's work, psychologist Perry London (1964, 1986) wrote a scholarly broadside about the neglect of the moral domain in the major models of psychotherapy. In a book clearly ahead of its time, *The Modes and Morals of Psychotherapy*, London was the first "insider" in the psychotherapy field to argue that the major models of therapy have implicit moral codes, most of which are about the primacy of individual agency to experience the life a person wants to live. For what he called "insight therapies" (e.g., Freudian, Rogerian, existential), social roles are external to the individual; they are chosen or discarded, as opposed to being core elements of what it means to be a person. Although relationships, of course, are important for individual development and happiness in all models of therapy, London (1986) observed that insight theorists "say that sociality is good for self, but they don't say how the good self, once fulfilled, is good for society" (p. 87).

London's book stood out because the entire vast literature on ethics and psychotherapy had dealt almost exclusively with the ethical practice of therapists in their professional role. Later exceptions that dealt with ethical issues in the lives of clients are Lageman (1993), Nichols (1994), Richardson et al. (1999), Peteet (2004), and more recently, Davis et al. (2021). Like London, these authors offered insights into the moral dimensions of therapy. However, their focus was not on the specifics of how to practice ethical consultation with clients (a goal of this book). In the field of family therapy, Ivan Boszormenyi-Nagy based his "contextual therapy" model on the concept of justice and intergenerational ethics (Boszormenyi-Nagy & Krasner, 1986). In addition, Fowers (2005) insightfully used virtue ethics to critique psychotherapy for ignoring moral agency, character, and moral commitments. He proposed "social goals" for therapy beyond the recovery or healing of the individual clients, goals that include stakeholders such as the client's family, social network, community, and even the larger society (Fowers et al., 2015). I return to this theme later in the book.

Backing up to my own earlier work, I argued in my 1995 book *Soul Searching: Why Psychotherapy Must Promote Moral Responsibility* that therapists in the first century of the field may have felt they could afford to ignore the ethical realm because they could assume that clients came with an overly rigid moral code

(Doherty, 1995). The job of the therapist was to help them find an authentic self in the midst of conventional prescriptions for behavior. For example, when divorce was rare and stigmatized, a therapist could assume that the client took marital commitment seriously and then focus on the other side of the ethical dilemma: the need of self for a satisfying relationship. This point echoes James Q. Wilson (1993), a public policy scholar, who noted the historical context of Freud and other early 20th century intellectuals and artists who rejected conventional morality: "[They] could take the product of a strong family life . . . [and good conduct] . . . for granted and get on with the task of liberating individuals from stuffy conventions, myopic religion, and political error" (p. 15).

What may have seemed appropriate for the early decades of psychotherapy became a poor fit later. By the time psychotherapy went mainstream in the last 3 decades of the 20th century, the culture was vastly different from the world of "stuffy conventions" blindly adhered to. Personal freedom was the mantra, along with political and cultural changes in the direction of emancipation from traditional restraints (Berkowitz, 2006). A popular wedding vow substituted the traditional "until death do us part" promise with the phrase "as long as we both shall love." The famous Gestalt Therapy Prayer penned by Fritz Perls (1969) showed up at wedding ceremonies I attended:

> I do my thing, and you do your thing.
> I am not in this world to live up to your expectations,
> And you are not in this world to live up to mine.
> You are you and I am I,
> And if by chance we find each other, it's beautiful.
> If not, it can't be helped. (p. 4)

Given the reach of the movement toward personal liberation, a pendulum swing was inevitable. Even Rollo May, the prominent existentialist psychologist and public intellectual, whose early writings indicted inauthentic living by conventional social roles and obligations, was reevaluating the role of psychotherapy by the 1990s:

> We in America have become a society devoted to the individual self. The danger is that psychotherapy becomes a self-concern, fitting . . . a new kind of client . . . the narcissistic personality. . . . We have made of therapy a new kind of cult, a method in which we hire someone to act as a guide to our successes and happiness. Rarely does one speak of duty to one's society. Almost everyone undergoing therapy is concerned with individual gain, and the psychotherapist is hired to assist in this endeavor. (May, 1992, p. xxv)

Despite these calls for a rebalancing of psychotherapy from an individualistic perspective to a more relational, contextual one, I believe that we have not advanced far, in part because we lack a detailed, clinically grounded road map for engaging with clients in an ethically sensitive way—sensitive to both the ethical domain of clients' lives and the ethics of our profession.

SHIFTING FROM INDIVIDUALISM TO A RELATIONAL FOCUS

In this book, I show how it's possible to respect the autonomy of clients while engaging them in therapeutic conversation about how they can balance their personal needs (self-interest) with their sense of responsibility to and for others. Two fundamental assumptions of this book are (a) humans are fundamentally moral and ethical beings in relational webs of mutual responsibility from birth to death and (b) that, like it or not, therapists are ethical consultants to our clients. But lacking an articulated framework for this ethical consultation work, most therapists just make it up as they go, generally defaulting to an individualistic orientation ("What do you need to do for you?") that downplays the role of responsibilities and obligations to others and community.

To engage in moral consultation, therapists do not have to dictate moral rules or claim to have all the answers. Rather, our role is not so different from how sociologist Alan Wolfe (1989) described the role of the social scientist when dealing with moral issues: "to locate a sense of moral obligation in common sense, ordinary emotions, and everyday life. . . . to help individuals discover and apply for themselves the moral rules they already, as social beings, possess" (pp. 214–215). Although many moral philosophers and some moral psychologists engage in hypothetical (and sometimes strange) ethical dilemmas to tease out ethical general principles, there is nothing esoteric about the ethical challenges discussed in this book: family commitments, fidelity versus affairs, truth telling versus lying, self-interest versus harming others, and obligations as citizens. A fundamental premise is that because clients don't separate the psychological and ethical aspects of their lives—"What am I feeling" is not separated from "What should I do?"—we owe it to them to become more skilled at ethical consultation.

This book draws inspiration from my 1995 book, *Soul Searching* (it's almost completely rewritten). My own journey on ethical consultation began a decade earlier when, in 1985, I read the landmark book *Habits of the Heart: Individualism and Commitment in American Life* (Bellah et al., 1985). I still remember how troubled I felt as I read this book's sections on psychotherapy as a cultural force. The authors argued that most psychotherapists were unwittingly promoting a form of "expressive individualism," which is a cousin of "utilitarian individualism." Utilitarian individualism, which they saw dominating political culture in the United States, is the idea that if individuals are free to pursue their private economic self-interest, the whole society will benefit. (Hence, there is little need to attend to the welfare of society as a whole.) Expressive individualism follows the same logic in the area of emotional well-being: Focus on yourself and the well-being of your family and community will follow.

The *Habits of the Heart* critique changed my view of therapy. I always knew that we are sometimes ineffective as therapists, but I had never considered the possibility that we could contribute to a cultural ethos that might erode two central elements of psychological health: commitment and community. It's not easy for any group of professionals to absorb how in doing our good work, we can harm the cultural environment. I recall presenting this critique at a workshop for therapists and being challenged by a participant who argued that women have been asked too often to sacrifice their personal goals for the benefit of others. "Isn't the most important gift a mother can give her daughters," she argued, "the role model of a woman pursuing her dreams?" Before I could respond, another participant raised her hand and blurted out, "That's exactly what my mother said as she left our family." Obviously thrown, the original speaker immediately qualified her previous remark, "Oh, I don't mean pursuing your dreams by abandoning your responsibilities." Here were the two sides of the tension between personal dreams and moral responsibilities. The first audience member who spoke up was not wrong but was articulating just one side of the tension—that of personal pursuit—without explicit consideration of who else is affected. The other audience member reminded her of the ethical context of personal choice. In everyday life, choosing between personal needs and moral responsibilities is a both/and—rather than an either/or—situation, but sometimes they are in tension.

Connected with this critique of therapeutic individualism was Bellah and colleagues' (1985) observation that therapy lacked a language of ethical or moral responsibility—a way to think and talk about commitments and responsibilities to others that cannot be translated and reduced to "What do I need to do for me?" In my training, we were taught to immediately challenge clients when they used the language of "ought" or "should," and we would have been confronted by our supervisors if we had introduced such ethical language. If "I should" could not be immediately translated into "I need" or "I want," it was considered inauthentic and unhealthy. If *Habits of the Heart* challenged me to see how my profession could be part of the problem in society, the challenge was what to do about it. How do we change in our everyday practice of therapy? There I had little guidance from the therapy literature.

My clinical turning point came with a client I will call Bruce, a 40ish-year-old man whose wife, Elaine, had just ended their marriage.[2] I had worked with them as a couple in the past. Bruce returned from work one day to find that Elaine had tossed his belongings into his car and changed the locks on the house. Overwhelmed and depressed, Bruce called me for a session. When we met, he told me he couldn't face the thought of going back to his house to pick up his children, a 3-year-old and a 6-year-old, for a visit. Even more intolerable was the prospect of returning alone to his small apartment after bringing them back to their mother. Tearfully, he said that he could not interact with Elaine after what she had done to him, although he still loved her and wanted to salvage their marriage. To compound matters, he had been fired from his job because he had not been showing up at work.

The more Bruce talked, the more he began to sprinkle in comments such as, "Maybe the kids would be better off if I just stayed away," and "I think I might need a complete break; maybe I should just pack up and move far away. There is nothing keeping me here now." In fact, a decade earlier, Bruce had given up contact with a child he had fathered with a woman he did not marry. Now that he had no job, the prospect of "starting all over somewhere else" was appealing to him.

I felt dismayed when he talked about abandoning his children, but my training had only equipped me with responses such as, "What do you need to do for yourself right now to get through this?" The most challenging statements from the traditional therapy paradigm I could offer a client like Bruce would be something such as, "I wonder whether you have considered the regret you will feel if you take yourself out of your children's lives," or "You may not be in a healthy enough frame of mind right now to make long-term decisions." There is nothing wrong with these statements; I used them in my conversation with Bruce. But I also decided to do something decidedly non-traditional: to challenge him in ethical terms. After listening to his pain over the end of his marriage and his desire to start over somewhere else, I asked him the kind of question considered out of bounds in my training: "How do you think it will affect your kids if you leave their lives?" He answered, "I think it will bother them for a while, but they'll get over it before long." I moved into deeper water by saying, "I think it will affect them for a long time, not just a short time. I'm concerned about them." Bruce was listening. His reply—"I'm worried about that too, but what kind of father will I be if I am an emotional wreck?"—gave me an opening.

---

[2]The description of this case is from "I'm O.K., You're O.K., but What About the Kids?," by W. J. Doherty, 1993, *The Family Therapy Networker, 17*, pp. 46–53. Copyright 1993 by the Family Therapy Network. Adapted with permission.

Throughout the conversation that ensued, I emphasized how important he was to them, even if he didn't think so right now and even if he was not emotionally at his best. I told him I could certainly understand that he might need a short time-out to collect himself before going back to his old house and facing his wife again. But he was irreplaceable to his children, and in my judgment, they would carry a lifelong emotional burden if he simply disappeared from their lives. Finally, I reminded him that his children were not responsible for the marital breakup and that it was not fair that they should be its casualties. I made these points not in the form of a lecture but as perspectives and opinions I offered as the conversation unfolded and Bruce pondered his course of action.

I'm sure that I am not the first therapist to respond this way to clients in similar situations. We do what we feel we have to do in crisis situations. Yet, I was struck by how little clinical training I had received on the moral and ethical issues I was confronting with Bruce, and I had good teachers. What mainstream theory of psychotherapy could I look to for support? Although I was trained as a family therapist to consider the multiple perspectives of family members, as a practical matter, family therapists can lose sight of the ethical stakeholders who are not present in therapy sessions. Like individual therapists, family therapists are comfortable talking about what clients need and deserve from other family members, but they are reluctant to talk about what clients owe other family members in care, commitment, fairness, or honesty.

To some therapists, my feedback to Bruce about his parental commitment may sound starkly moralistic, but I wanted to make two things clear to him: I was not neutral on his decision about staying committed to his children, and I was giving priority to his children's long-term needs over his short-term distress. Bruce, with whom I had a bond of trust, grasped my point and quickly moved from *whether* to stay involved to *how* to accomplish it. In the end, he remained a committed father and later reconnected with his child from the previous relationship.

When I described this case to my colleagues, some suggested that I could have obtained the same result—Bruce staying involved with his children—by just emphasizing the remorse he would eventually feel if he abandoned them. I did use these appeals because I think they are valid. Parents' relationships with their children can be deeply rewarding; when a parent abandons a child, the parent too is damaged. However, in dealing with ethical decisions I think it is generally a mistake to appeal only to a client's self-interest (even if that appeal "works") because the ethic of personal gain removed from the ethic of responsible commitment erodes the quality of our clients' lives and ultimately the quality of community life. And practically speaking, what would I say next if Bruce indicated that he could handle the remorse and maybe have more children in the future? In some situations where the client is blind to how they may be harming others, we have to be willing to go beyond appeals to self-interest.

After I made these points during a workshop, a therapist in the audience approached me with her story. She used to feel comforted when her therapist husband would say that he was committed to being sexually faithful to her not because it was wrong or would hurt her, but because it would hurt him—by violating his integrity. He couldn't live with himself, he maintained, if he broke his promise by having an affair. The wife told me that this kind of commitment felt good because it seemed so internalized and authentic—until her husband had an affair and left her for a younger woman. He apparently decided that he could live with himself after all.

To repeat, expanding the therapeutic conversation beyond the client's self-interest pushes most therapists past our training and beyond most psychotherapy literature. In most models of therapy, the lingua franca is self-speak: I want, I need, I feel, I think. Even those who also speak "systems" tend to appeal to individuals in terms of personal needs and desires. Again, I am not saying that being concerned with clients' needs is an invalid therapeutic concern. I am arguing that when that becomes our only consideration, therapy lacks moral and human depth, and therapists end up promoting a kind of trickle-down psychological economics. Nor am I suggesting that behind closed doors there are no other therapists who address ethical issues. But because we lack a conscious moral tradition that can be discussed, debated, and refined, we are left to make it up as we go.

After working with Bruce on his commitment as a father, I was changed as a therapist. I began to see more times when ethical issues are wrapped up with clinical issues. I became more aware of how I had previously promoted an ethical agenda of self-interest without being conscious of it. For the first time, I began translating the insights of social scientists such as Robert Bellah to my everyday work with clients.

Later, when I wrote *Soul Searching*, I articulated a model for how therapists can engage in what I called "moral consultation" with clients in a way that expanded the purview of what was possible to discuss in therapy. After it was published, I waited for a pushback that never came. Most therapists who read the book and heard me speak about it did not quarrel with the idea that we are not value neutral and that we tend to be individualistic, but I did not see much in the way of therapists changing how they think and practice. Twenty years later, however, I began to see new interest in U.S.

therapists in interpersonal ethics and social justice, perhaps because our culture has changed. (A cultural marker of mainstream cultural interest in ethics is *The New York Times* column "The Ethicist" that was inaugurated in 1999 and continues to be popular in the 2020s.) The ethical domain is more in the public conversation, and we therapists are changing with the larger culture.

When I finished *Soul Searching*, I knew that the most conceptually unfinished chapter was the one on community. Nowadays, it's hard to ignore the public or community dimensions of therapy when issues of political polarization, social justice, racial reconciliation, and public health crises invade the therapist's office. I also find myself better able than in the 1990s to articulate the connection between the personal sphere and the civic sphere because so much of my work in the past 2 decades has been in the area of civic engagement and democracy building. I pick up this theme in Chapter 8. The ethics of everyday life is not only about the intimate sphere, but it's also about our roles as citizens of larger communities.

OVERVIEW OF THE BOOK

As mentioned, most prior writing on the topic of this book has focused on the conceptual level as opposed to articulating how to do ethical consultation with a wide range of issues that clients present. Because I want this book to be useful to practicing therapists, students, and teachers, it will be intensely case oriented after Chapter 1, which lays out theory and research underlying my approach. In terms of that chapter, since I published *Soul Searching*, there has been quite a lot of recent scholarship on the social psychology of morality.

Chapter 2 begins the clinical application by laying out a number of basic skills in what I call "ethical consultation" in therapy. Some of these skills look like the everyday craft of therapy—listening, exploring, affirming, and offering perspective—as applied to situations when clients bring their ethical concerns to therapy sessions. The more advanced skill of ethical challenge most often comes into play when the therapist sees an ethical issue that clients don't see themselves.

Chapter 3 begins the set of chapters on application to specific ethical concerns and dilemmas. The first issue is commitments: keeping and breaking them. Chapter 4 deals with affairs in a different way from the current literature because it discusses clients currently having an affair. In Chapter 5, I address how clients deal with their experience of lying, deceiving, and secret keeping—again, something the literature typically addresses in terms of how clients are impacted by the deceit of others in their lives rather than how they deal with their own choices in this domain. Chapter 6 directly takes on situations of harm that clients might be causing others, including intended and unintended emotional, psychological, and physical harm; most current literature deals with this issue in the relatively uncommon situation of the ethical and legal duty to warn a third party about a threat of violence (Felthous, 2006). These chapters are case oriented with practical guidelines based on the LEAP-C framework of skills.

Chapter 7 addresses the self of the therapist in ethical consultation, with a focus on both personal and cultural levels. In the individualist culture out of which psychotherapy was born, we imagine that we are being value free and morally neutral when supporting a client to mainly emphasize self-interest in the face of an ethical dilemma (if you are not happy in the marriage, why are you staying?). The ethical self of the therapist moves us into cultural self-awareness as well as personal self-awareness. Chapter 8 explores the role of therapists in sustaining and advancing civic life and democratic engagement in an era of increasing disconnection and political polarization. The book concludes with an Afterword that highlights two cautionary tales involving public figures involved in high-profile scandals—Woody Allen and Monica Lewinski—whose psychotherapists did not offer them moral consultation. These examples demonstrate that psychotherapists' responsibilities extend beyond their clients to others they interact with and to the wider public. In that regard, I still feel challenged by a book I read decades ago: *We've Had a Hundred Years of Psychotherapy—And the World's Getting Worse* (Hillman & Ventura, 1993). I believe that if we can "crack the code" on how to be skilled, sensitive, and intentional about addressing ethical issues in therapy, we can not only better help our clients but also contribute to building a more connected and just world.

PART I THE SCIENCE AND PRACTICE OF ETHICAL CONSULTATION

1 FOUNDATIONS OF ETHICAL CONSULTATION IN THERAPY

Although the psychotherapy literature has paid little attention to the ethical world of clients, in recent decades, social psychology has seen a blossoming of theory and research in this area. When I wrote *Soul Searching* in the 1990s, the prevailing models were heavily cognitive, emphasizing moral reasoning (Kohlberg, 1984). I found this cognitive approach, with its focus on reasoning about hypothetical moral dilemmas, not especially useful for psychotherapy. The state of more applicable psychological theory and research in the early 21st century is illustrated by the no less than 57 chapters written by a variety of scholars in Gray and Graham's (2018) volume *Atlas of Moral Psychology*. It's noteworthy, however, that the index contains not a single reference to psychotherapy.

In this chapter, I offer moral foundations theory (Haidt & Joseph, 2007) and social constructionism (Meade, 1956) as a theoretical basis for ethical consultation in therapy. I present preliminary data from therapists about the kinds of ethical concerns their clients bring to therapy. And because I don't believe that ethical consultation can be simply grafted onto traditional individualistic views of the self, I outline a way of thinking about the relational self that inherently involves interpersonal commitments.

https://doi.org/10.1037/0000263-002
The Ethical Lives of Clients: Transcending Self-Interest in Psychotherapy, by W. J. Doherty

MORAL FOUNDATIONS THEORY

The main reasons I find Haidt's moral foundation theory useful are its focus on moral intuitions and emotions, its empirical base in cross-cultural research, and its applicability to social and political controversies (Haidt, 2012; Haidt & Joseph, 2007). This model came out of three streams of research: cultural anthropological studies of morality, evolutionary psychology, and the work of Kahneman (2017) and others on automatic thinking (Graham et al., 2018). For our purposes, its main principle is that "intuitions come first." Moral judgments happen quickly and are influenced heavily by emotion: For the most part, we quickly intuit moral judgments and then explain them rationally afterward. These responses constitute "the moral mind," which develops over time for individuals within a culture. Moral foundations theory posits that cultural intuitions in the form of moral foundations are adaptive responses to the social challenges humans have faced during evolutionary history. Our success as a species has depended on working out ways to cooperate as social animals in different environments.

The following moral foundations are the ones most well established in research conducted by Haidt and his colleagues. Although they are found in all cultures studied thus far, the foundations are emphasized differently in varied cultures (Haidt & Joseph, 2007). I describe these foundations and illustrate them by examples that show up in therapy.

- *Care/harm* is related to attachment systems and our ability to feel and dislike the pain of others. This domain comes up in therapy in relation to clients' responsibilities for caregiving and managing relationships where there is attachment and vulnerability.

- *Fairness/cheating* is related to reciprocal altruism and the ideas of justice, rights, and autonomy. It comes up in therapy in regard to issues such as lying and secret keeping as well as sexual infidelity.

- *Loyalty/betrayal* is related to our history in tribes and coalition building. It underlies virtues such as patriotism and sacrifice for the group. It comes up in therapy in issues such as obligations to spouse versus family of origin, divided loyalties in stepfamilies, and differences in group allegiances (e.g., religious, political) that can create conflicts among family members.

- *Authority/subversion* is based on our human history with hierarchy. This underlies the virtues of leadership and followership and respect for traditions. It surfaces in therapy in regard to coparenting differences in discipline, conflict over respect for family elders and traditions, and family differences over following religious and political leaders.

- *Purity/degradation* relates to disgust and contamination connected to the body and religious notions of striving to be elevated and less carnal. This comes up in issues related to sexuality and religion.

These five constructs, which have some overlap among them, can serve as a guide for therapists when listening for the intuitions at play for clients when they face ethical dilemmas. Laura, the adult daughter trying to find a way to continue to offer support for a difficult mother as described in the Introduction, was dealing with moral intuitions related to care/harm and loyalty/betrayal, which were in tension with her personal needs.[1] Her mother had no other family to care for her as she aged, and my client did not feel right about the advice of her friends to abandon her caregiving obligations to her mother. The goal of my ethical consultation was for the client to find a way to maintain her own well being while acting in accord with her moral intuitions.

According to moral foundations researchers, highly educated individuals in Western culture, particularly those of a relatively liberal political persuasion, tend to use only the first two moral constructs: care/harm and fairness/cheating (Haidt, 2012). In fact, the other ethical bases are somewhat suspect because they reflect a more collectivist view of human beings. Doing something because of, say, authority or tradition bumps up against the liberal cultural norm of individual authenticity. I am probably correct in speculating that the great majority of therapists are in this liberal, individualistic camp. If so, moral intuitions based on domains such as authority, loyalty, and purity are more difficult for many therapists to understand and appreciate than intuitions based on harm or unfairness to specific other people.

Skepticism about some of the moral foundations could make it difficult for a therapist to work with clients from other cultures. I felt this challenge when working with an Iranian immigrant couple who came to see me for help in making their 18-year-old son, who had come out to them as gay, turn into a heterosexual. They were so ashamed that they took 30 minutes to tell me specifically what they thought was wrong with their son and how they wanted me to help. After I respectfully declined their request that I try to change their son's sexual orientation, they told me that they were considering cutting him out of their lives because of their religious belief in the evil of homosexuality.

I found myself thinking in terms of harm to their son, who was leaving home and moving to New York City for college during the height of the AIDS

---

[1]The case examples in this chapter have been modified to disguise the identities of the clients involved and to protect their confidentiality.

epidemic. Being cut off by his parents, I feared, could be devastating to him (their relationship apparently had been good before he came out) and put him at considerable risk as a newly out young man far from home. While my mind was initially focused on care/harm, the parents were emphasizing authority/subversion in terms of their allegiance to their religious tradition and perhaps loyalty to their Muslim community. I sensed that setting up a conflict between harm and authority would be a nonstarter in my consultation with them. I had to find a way to work with both moral intuitions.

My ethical consultation focused first on affirming their deep love for their son, without which they would not be agonizing over their decision, and then on their worry about compromising their deeply held religious beliefs if they accepted their son and his sexual orientation. Once I sensed that they felt heard and affirmed, I expressed my concern about the great risk to their son at this point in his life if he were to lose them, and then without pausing, I expressed the other side of their dilemma, namely, that protecting their son from harm felt like abandoning their deeply felt religious beliefs. Note that if I had paused after my expression of concern about harm to their son, without immediately articulating the other moral intuition at stake, they could easily have responded with a "yes, but," arguing the side of their dilemma I had not yet articulated. In Chapter 2, I discuss this kind of microskill in ethical consultation.

Haidt's moral foundations theory is not without critics who see it as underplaying the role of moral reasoning (Narvaez, 2010) and as unsophisticated in terms of neurobiological underpinnings of moral foundations (Suhler & Churchland, 2011). Nor are the five foundations a checklist for therapists to run through. But they can provide a sensitizing map for listening to and respecting a client's moral intuitions and the tensions among them. And in a culture of expressive individualism, they can help us avoid the temptation to ignore or devalue moral emotions and intuitions that are important for many clients in a pluralistic society. Chapter 7 goes into more detail about cultural issues in ethical consulting.

THE PRIMACY OF HARM IN ETHICAL CONSULTATION

Let's return to my working definition of the moral/ethical domain for ethical consultation by therapists: client behavior that has consequences for the welfare of others. If moral foundations theory posits at least five universal moral intuitions, how can I justify a focus that seems to entertain just one category—care/harm (which is the core dimension of "welfare of others")?

For one reason, in responding to critics who say that all moral foundations come down to care/harm, Haidt and his colleagues admit that

> If you had to pick one foundation as the most important single one, in terms of both importance and prototypicality, care/harm is probably the best candidate. Evidence has been shown for the centrality, ubiquity, and prototypicality of harm in (negative) moral judgments. (Graham et al., 2018, p. 215)

Beyond this centrality in the research, it is plausible that there is a harm dimension in all the other moral foundations, given that morality has emerged in human communities to safeguard the well-being of the people in those communities. Even most purity codes were probably developed to protect people from bad outcomes, as seen at the time. Similarly, loyalty and respect for authority maintain solidarity and social norms that protect community members from harm. And, of course, fairness and cheating directly affect care and harm for individuals and communities.

Having made the argument for the centrality of care/harm in ethical consultation, I don't want to fall into the Western, individualist trap of saying that the other moral foundations are not useful for the therapist to keep in mind and affirm for clients. But for purposes of ethical consultation by therapists in a pluralistic society, there is merit in emphasizing the avoidance of harm to people affected by our client's actions. This is particularly important when the therapist decides to challenge the client on ethical grounds when the client is not expressing an ethical concern (as in my work with Bruce described in the Introduction). If I am going to challenge clients' blind spots in the ethical domain, I'd better be on firm ground. I believe that avowing harm to others does represent the closest thing we have in a pluralistic society to firm ground as a moral norm. Witness the ubiquity of the Golden Rule, stated in one form as "whatever you do not want someone to do to you, do not do it to them." The ethic of not harming others is behind the interpersonal prohibitions in the Ten Commandments—do not lie, steal, commit adultery, or murder—as well as the positive commandment to honor your parents (which no doubt reflected for adults the importance of not letting harm befall them).

In contrast, if I were to challenge a client's ethical behavior on the basis of, say, respect for authority or tradition, I would be on shakier grounds. As a secular therapist in a pluralistic society, I would be reluctant to raise an ethical concern about clients not following their respected authorities or traditions. Note the differences between *exploring* a client's ambivalence about following a religious mandate versus *challenging* the client's thinking or actions based on the tradition's claims. (Challenging clients is something I am willing to do if a third party is being harmed.) This might be different for a pastoral counselor working with someone who came for help because of a shared religious tradition. But for most therapists in a pluralistic culture, I believe it's best to privilege interpersonal morality related to avoiding harm—is someone getting hurt here? To be clear, though, a therapist should be able to explore the meaning of all the moral foundations for clients.

WHAT ETHICAL ISSUES DO CLIENTS BRING TO THERAPY?

I know of no research on which client ethical issues come up in therapy. However, I have polled several hundred therapists who have taken my workshops on ethical consultation in therapy. During the first morning of the workshop, after I describe what I mean by the ethical dimension of client's lives and the five moral foundations from Haidt's work, I give participants a sheet of paper with these directions:

> Please briefly describe an example or two of an ethical issue in the life of a client that you found challenging to address therapeutically. It could be something that the client brought to you or something that you saw but was not an issue raised by the client.

Exhibit 1.1 presents an informal categorization of the responses. As you will see, most fall under the umbrella of client actions or decisions that can potentially cause harm. The major categories are secret keeping, divorce decisions, dangerous or illegal behaviors, parent behaviors related to risk for children, and a variety of actions that create safety risks for others. The therapists were asked to write a paragraph about the challenges they faced in handling these situations. Mostly they reported feeling unprepared and inadequate, especially when it came to challenging a client about potentially harmful behavior the client did not see as problematic.

To conclude this section on care/harm as a focus for ethical consultation, note that simply identifying the ethical issues does not make it easy to discern the path forward. For example, the ethic of caring for and not harming one's frail parents could lead, in one culture or life circumstance, to placement in a nursing home instead of taking the parents into one's home, while in another culture or circumstance, say with poor placement facilities, such a placement could be seen as harmful abandonment. Certainly, decisions about divorce are fraught with complexities. Neither the therapist nor the client has to know the "right" path to take to explore possible paths in an ethically sensitive way that balances the needs of self with responsibilities to others.

EXHIBIT 1.1. Client Ethical Dilemmas From Workshop Participants

Secrets

- Affairs (past and ongoing)
- Intent to divorce/leave relationship, not telling spouse
- Abortions
- Limits on how long to keep secrets
- About the biological mother
- Pornography use

Divorce

- Kids
- Financial security
- Spouse's physical or mental illness
- Ambivalence

Illegal or dangerous behavior

- Cheating on taxes
- Past crimes (e.g., murder, sexual abuse)
- Substance abuse during pregnancy
- Drinking and driving

Parents and child safety

- Fitness to parent
- Client denying responsibility for child sexual abuse or not believing child's accusations
- Sexually active minor
- Child not in school
- Parental threats to abandon

Others' safety

- Spreading sexually transmitted diseases
- Young or vulnerable sexual partners
- Systemic impact of client's unhealthy behavior
- Working with a pedophile client

THE SOCIAL CONSTRUCTION OF ETHICAL CHOICES IN THERAPY

One other conceptual framework complements moral foundations theory, with a focus on how ethical choices emerge in current social interactions: the social constructionist model coming out of the work of early 20th-century sociologist George Herbert Meade (1956) and other scholars who emphasized "the social construction of reality" (Berger & Luckmann, 1966). (Alan Wolfe's, 1989, work described in the Introduction comes out of that tradition.) In this theoretical perspective, morality is created and modified through social interaction, beginning in childhood and continuing into adulthood. We are in continual social interaction, storytelling, and conversation about what we and the people around us, including political figures and celebrities, are doing that is right or wrong. It's the stuff of everyday gossip about someone's affair, as well deeper deliberation on whether a war is justified.

From this perspective, psychotherapy is a specialized form of conversation, a social interaction where clients share their meanings and emotions, including ethical ones, in a flow of dialogue with the therapist. Clients don't deliver up their ethical dilemmas for us to evaluate and advise them on. They tell us what's troubling them and we help them navigate a central tension in the human experience: the sometimes-competing needs of self and others. As I've argued, we don't have a choice about engaging in this role if we are open to clients bringing in their real-world ethical struggles and dilemmas. We either do our ethical consultation well—with theory, research, and skills to guide us—or we do it willy-nilly, likely guided by the expressive individualistic ethic of a consumer culture. This point bears repeating with emphasis: To claim to be value free in work with clients is to be under the influence of the mainstream value orientation of one's culture.

TOWARD A NEW VIEW OF THE RELATIONAL SELF IN ETHICALLY INFORMED THERAPY[2]

As Rieff (1966) and London (1986) pointed out decades ago, underlying every therapy model are assumptions about what it means to be a human being, a self, at a specific historical and cultural moment. During the 20th century, psychotherapy was a prominent shaper of the cultural image of the self. During the first half of the century, an era with two world wars, large-scale social change, and discontent among intellectuals, psychoanalytic theory espoused the complex/conflicted self, an inner personal world of ambivalence, contradiction, and sublimated desires. Psychotherapy helped clients understand and accept their conflicted needs and desires, including socially unacceptable ones, with the goal of an integrated sense of self that is never fully free of contradictions, such as loving and hating the same people. The human journey comes with never-resolved dialectics of attachment and fear of dependency, responsibility and self-indulgence, and insight and self-delusion. This view of the self aptly fit the Western world in the middle third of the 20th century, when psychoanalysis flowered in psychotherapy

---

[2]Portions of this section are adapted from Doherty (2020a).

and influenced cultural elites (Zaretsky, 2005). It was an era of survival and living with limits.

The post–World War II economic boom and the rise of an educated middle class brought on a new era: the social liberation movements of the 1960s (Steigerwald, 1995). In response to a new cultural environment, new therapies emerging from the human potential movement promoted immediate change that did not require years of archeological exploration of the human psyche. They offered a new image of the self: the liberated/authentic self, self-determining, self-actualizing, and not stifled by social conformity. Social historians have documented how humanistic psychotherapy grew out of 1960s culture and, in turn, contributed to a new ideal of the free-to-be-you-and-me self (Anderson, 2004).

But as the human potential movement faded, there came a reckoning with the idea of the liberated/authentic self. By the 1980s and 1990s, it looked unbalanced, too self-absorbed, and too free to manipulate others for self-gratification. It also ignored multiculturalism and institutional forms of oppression that were now coming into the public conversation in an increasingly polarized society (Gerstle, 2017). Unfortunately, the therapy world did not offer a new model of the self to replace the liberated/authentic self. Therapists in the late 20th century were coming to grips with managed care and the medical model. They were working on newly recognized problems such as trauma and attachment injuries, and they were trying to gain a foothold in the marketplace via evidence-based legitimacy. Although this was important internal work, it was not on the cutting edge of cultural change. Bestseller lists that once were headed by therapists were turned over to media celebrities and business authors.

The Consumer Self

As therapists attended our knitting, a new cultural image of the self took hold: the consumer self. As described by the sociologist Lizabeth Cohen (2008) in her book *Consumer America*, the consumer culture had been growing since the end of World War II, when the U.S. government asked Americans to ward off a potential economic downturn (there were fears of a return to the Great Depression) by spending their money on consumer goods. This spending contributed to an unprecedented economic boom during which millions of Americans moved into the middle class and were eager to keep spending their resources. This economic phenomenon influenced cultural values: A popular saying of the 1980s was "The one who dies with the most toys wins." In fact, according to Cohen, the consumer culture tends to colonize all spheres of society. Thus, the antimaterialistic youth of the

Human Potential Movement went from singing "All You Need Is Love" to writing commercial jingles. Tony Robbins replaced Carl Rogers. Business leaders appropriated Maslow's hierarchy of needs.

The consumer self, of course, is ultimately an empty self. The toys lose their pleasures, and there is always someone with more of them. There is always someone with more status and prestige in a hypercompetitive society. Virtually unlimited choice turns out not to be liberating but anxiety inducing as consumers feel anxious about whether they made the "right" choice (Murphy, 2016). The consumer self, it turns out, is at risk of social isolation, insecurity, and the lure of tribalism when leaders tell people that their unhappiness comes from the other taking advantage of them.

Personal relationships too become more fragile in a consumer culture because their main source is not lasting commitment or enduring friendship but the sense of whether the relationship is "working for me" these days. Even the desire to do well by those we love can become caught up in consumerism, as witnessed by how middle-class parenting is becoming a competition to help their children make it in a society where economic success is the highest form of accomplishment (Doherty, 2000). In some urban areas, the competition begins with exams to enter high-status preschools.

At a civic level, the consumer culture accelerated the decline in civic engagement. Long gone was John F. Kennedy's call to national service, replaced on the political right by promises to tax less and on the left by promises of more government services. Participation in the "civil society" (voluntary associations), which involves both contributing and receiving, continued a perilous decline that had begun in the 1960s, as documented in Robert Putnam's (2001) classic book *Bowling Alone*. Putnam (2020) updated and vastly expanded his analysis of American society in his book *The Upswing*. Analyzing empirical data from the past 140 years, he painted a picture of a society moving from the hyperindividualism of the Gilded Age (the robber baron, no safety net, social Darwinist era of the late 20th century) to the more collectivist era of the mid-20th century (the reform-oriented Progressive Era, the New Deal, the mutual sacrifices of World War II, the solidarity-against-communism era of the 1950s). Then, according to Putnam, we returned to a more individualistic culture beginning in the 1960s and accelerating thereafter with globalization, hypercompetitiveness, and levels of income inequality not seen since the late 19th century. In Putnam's summary phrase, we went "from I to we to I." Commenting on the era we are currently in, Putnam (2020) wrote,

> As the 1960s moved into the 1970s, 1980s, and beyond, we re-created the socioeconomic chasm of the last Gilded Age at an accelerated pace. In that same

period we replaced cooperation with political polarization. We allowed our community and family ties to unravel to a marked extent. And our culture became far more focused on individualism and less interested in the common good. (p. 11)

My central argument in this book is that the field of psychotherapy was influenced by and contributed to this cultural trend toward too much "I" and that we can now help create a healthier balance between the I and the we—between the individual and the communal. But this can only occur if we admit to being part of the problem we aim to fix.

The Individualistic, Consumer Self in Therapy

I began to see the consumer self in therapy during the 1980s. Clients who were unhappy in their marriage now added something like "This isn't the deal I signed up for up for when I got married." Therapy colleagues told me they would ask clients whether a problem was a "deal breaker" for them in their marriage—and they weren't referring to abuse or chronic affairs. Marriage in a consumer culture becomes transactional like other relationships—what you do for me and I do for you.

The fragility of transactional, consumer relationships even shows up in parenting. The head of a shelter and treatment house, founded in the 1960s for "runaway youth," told me that by the 1990s, the biggest client category was not runaway kids but "throwaway kids." Many didn't get along with mom's or dad's new partner, and it came down to who would be evicted. The new partner often won.

The first time I thought of a clinical case in terms of the consumer culture of parenting, it was with a depressed 14-year-old girl, Tobi, whose middle-class parents wanted to be more communicative.[3] The family had entered therapy over issues with a younger sibling who had a brain disorder, but in our sessions, Tobi soon became the focus of the parents' concerns. Tobi, I came to realize, was burdened by excessive expectations for her to provide care and disciplinary limits for her younger brother. Despite my efforts, the parents had trouble seeing how they had parentified her.

In a memorable family therapy session, the father complained about a family dinner that illustrated Tobi's refusal to communicate. When the parents asked Tobi about her day at school, she responded like a typical adolescent with a shrug and little information—at which point the father angrily sent her to her room: "If that's the attitude you are going to have, you can eat in your room by yourself." (The mother supported this reprimand and

---

[3]This case example is adapted from Doherty (2017c).

consequence.) During the session, Tobi sat silent and glum while her father recounted the story and then asked a question that chilled me: "How long do we have to keeping giving to this child before we can expect to get something in return?" The mother nodded her assent.

I had been a family therapist for many years but never faced a moment, or a comment, like this. I felt like screaming at the parents or scooping up the girl or both. Instead, I took a breath and addressed the parents slowly and intensely, holding back a vocal tremble that seemed to want to come out: "She's your daughter. You have to keep giving and giving. [Pause] What you can expect back is respect and cooperation but not openness with her feelings because that has to be a free gift." During a pause when the parents took this in, I saw Tobi sitting up in her chair. Fortunately, the father softened (I didn't have a follow-up move in mind!) and said, "I don't know how to reach her." I responded gently, "I think you do know how to reach her, and I can help." Time was over for the session.

During the week before our next session, I pushed myself to frame what happened not in terms of bad, uncaring parents (or assigning them more sophisticated labels), but instead, I thought of them as loving but unrealistic parents influenced by a consumer culture where disappointments and frustrations are processed via the lingua franca of self-interest: "What about my needs?" I was nervous about the next session because I knew I could not just repeat my "step up and be a parent" speech. The tone of the session was immediately different. Tobi was smiling and talkative. The parents said they had reflected a lot on the last session and reported that things had gone much better with Tobi. My voice choked up as I told the parents how much I admired them for their willingness to absorb a strong challenge from me in the last session. This was not a miracle cure. The family had a longer journey to walk, and it was not easy to get Tobi out of the parentified role, but the parents had let go of their entitlement with regard to Tobi, and she was no longer the focal point for their frustrated expectations for family harmony in the face of a challenging, disabled child.

Therapy and Cultural Influence

In recent years, therapists have been developing ways to treat the isolated consumer self: We've been emphasizing attachment and connection. But we have not regained cultural influence, in part, I believe, because we have confronted the ramifications of the me-first consumer culture and its image of the self. In contrast, early psychoanalysts offered a potent critique of the Victorian and post-Victorian culture of repression, and therapists in the Human Potential Movement identified and criticized the postwar culture of conformity that it sought to transcend.

To become culture influencers today will require looking not just at the personal problems we see in our offices but also at the cultural pathologies that underlie them. We've gone partway in that direction through a substantial literature on the problems of racism and poverty (e.g., McGoldrick & Hardy, 2008). But I believe that we are not also focusing on the forces of hyperindividualism, consumer materialism, and tribalization, which arguably are part of the reason for a recent decline in self-reported well-being in the U.S. population (Witters, 2017)—and which prevent us from addressing the communal problems of racism and poverty. As Putnam (2020) pointed out, individualistic cultures pull back from addressing communal issues.

Cultural influence requires an alternative to the status quo. In the 1960s and 1970s, the alternative was the liberated/authentic self. Today, I see the ingredients of a new ideal of the self. I see it in our field's best developments in recent decades. It's a vision of the relational self, with two core dimensions: connection and commitment (see also Doherty, 2020a).

The Relational Self

The relational self is more than the obvious idea that we all need relationships, and it's more than the interpersonal actions taken by an individual. It's a conceptual shift to seeing relationships not just as voluntary bonds that we take on or discard but as inherent in the very concept of the self. In other words, it's not an individualistic self having relationships but relationships as a core constituent of the self. Stated formally, there is no self-system outside of relational systems. Stated more informally, there is no I without a we. In making a similar point, Slife and Wiggins (2009), inspired by Buber (1958) and Levinas (1969), distinguished between a "weak" form of relational thinking in psychology—the individual in a set of relationships—to a "strong" form of relational thinking that views the self as "ontologically" constituted by relationships and responsibility to others in relationships. This has profound implications for how we view culture and society—and for the practice of psychotherapy

The idea of a relational self was a core principle of family systems theory that became obscured when family therapy entered the mainstream as an intervention to treat individual disorders in the *Diagnostic and Statistical Manual of Mental Disorders* (American Psychiatric Association, 2013). It's a centerpiece of interpersonal neurobiology (Siegel, 2015), contemporary attachment-oriented therapies (Johnson, 2013; Steele & Steele, 2018), and the development of relational psychoanalysis (Mitchell & Aron, 1999). Some identity theory literature in psychology explicitly uses the term "the relational self" (Chen et al., 2006), but the core idea predates modern psychology. The relational self resurrects the premodern notion (it's clear in Homer) that there is no fully separate self—we are big-brained bees in a hive—but with a modern emphasis on the complexity and agency of the individual person.

In the more we-oriented culture of the 1950s and early 1960s (Putnam, 2020), the founders of family therapy focused on the pathologies of together-ness: family enmeshment or fusion from which an individual needs to form a differentiated self. If family enmeshment was the modal problem of the mid-20th century, a greater concern today is whether relational bonds can hold at all. The enmeshed family has given way to the disengaged family, the conformist community where people are into your business, to the neighbor-hood where nobody knows your name (Putnam, 2020). If this perspective is accurate, we need more "gluing" interventions, not just the traditional personal agency interventions (although those are still important).

At the community and societal level, the idea of the relational self speaks to the importance of authentic connections across group differences (see Chapter 8). Without those relational bonds, people become isolated and in need of therapy. They are also drawn to false tribalism, such as pitting conservative "reds" and liberal "blues" against each other in everything from personal lifestyles to national politics (Hetherington & Weiler, 2018). We humans are relational and communitarian, and if either pole is unhealthy, the individual person is unhealthy.

Commitment and the Relational Self

But "relational" alone is not a strong enough idea to counteract the fragmen-tation of today's world. After all, relationships come and go. For this reason, I am placing the notion of commitment as a core element of the relational self. By "commitment," I mean sustained investment in something outside oneself, to relationships and causes that transcend us, extend us, challenge us, and require a continual struggle to manage and even sacrifice for (Doherty, 1995; Taylor, 1992). The importance of commitment comes from the fact that we are born into families and communities that both support us (even if imperfectly) and call on us to give back. In other words, these relationships come with ethical obligations to be sustained over time, even difficult times.

Ethical commitment is inconsistent with the consumer self that honors no previous obligations unless they promise future rewards. As law professor Tim Wu (2017) pointed out in his book *The Attention Merchants*, consumer capitalism is the most creative force in the contemporary world, able to trans-form any personal or collective ideal into a consumer desire. In the inter-personal realm, consumer culture promotes a sense of entitlement to the best possible relationships, preferably those with low maintenance and high rewards. Therefore, a new image of the relational self must include the ability to form lasting ethical commitments, or it will be subsumed by the transactional ethic of consumer culture. Why should I work at a relationship that's not working for me?

Historically, the therapy literature has not paid much attention to commitment. The literature on child and family therapy assumes but has not made explicit the idea that parents have obligations to their children that rise to the level of ethical commitment: A parent should not simply walk away from these obligations when they become difficult. (An exception is the intergenerational ethics approach of family therapy pioneer Ivan Boszormenyi-Nagy [Boszormenyi-Nagy & Krasner, 1986].) In the couples therapy field, there has been work on marital commitment and divorce, with almost all therapists agreeing that divorce is a necessary safety valve for some toxic marriages. But the agreement stops there in terms of whether couples therapists should be neutral about divorce or promote marital commitment when feasible (Doherty, 2015; Wall et al., 1999).

Recently, however, couple therapy leaders have been coalescing around the value of marital commitment (Stanley, 2005). John Gottman and Julie Gottman (2021), for example, have begun emphasizing the importance of commitment, which, they wrote,

> means believing (and acting on the belief) that your relationship with this person is completely your lifelong journey, for better or for worse (meaning that if it gets worse, you'll both work to improve it). It implies cherishing your partner's positive qualities and nurturing gratitude. (Commitment section)

Michele Weiner-Davis (2002) has long emphasized marital commitment; for a time, she was nearly alone in opposing therapist neutrality when it comes to divorce. Although the prominent attachment-based emotionally focused therapy does not employ commitment as a central term, proponents clearly promote enduring bonds of connection (Johnson, 2013). In that work, attachment requires a sense of commitment, which creates a safe space for vulnerability, and attachment, in turn, can foster greater commitment to repair a broken relationship. Chapter 3 addresses the ethical issue of commitment in more depth.

Community and the Public Dimensions of the Self

The relational self as I conceptualize it is communitarian. It is not limited to the intimate sphere because human beings exist in groups larger than family and close friends (Doherty, 2017c). Most traditional theories in psychotherapy have not paid much attention to articulate a public dimension of the self (there are exceptions, such as Adler, 1927/1992), which means there is little psychological guidance for how individuals and their families can be productive citizens in the larger world and its institutions. This gap is at the heart of concerns by social scientists about the contemporary retreat from broad social engagement and commitment to civic life (Bellah et al., 1985; Putnam, 2016). Marriages, families, and other close relationships must fulfill all the social needs of individuals—and often fail the task.

In this regard, here is a provocative but necessary question for therapists in the 21st century when democratic nations and communities are weakening: What roles can we play in sustaining and promoting democracy? By democracy, I don't mean only elections and government. I mean democracy as "collective agency," the capacity of people to work together to solve problems and create a common world in which to live. Democracy, in John Dewey's (1993) terms, is a way of life, not just a form of government. In the framing of Harry Boyte (2005), democracy is about "public work": ordinary people deliberating across differences and taking responsibility for their future together. In the 21st century, we have to think of this as a "multiracial democracy" that offers liberty, equality, and justice to all groups, with special consideration to include those groups who were outsiders in the creation of modern democratic nations.

To return to my question for therapists: What role can we play in a world where democracy as collective agency appears to be fragile and where subgroups within nations are increasingly polarized? This is a question pertinent to a particular moment of history, just as our predecessors posed questions about how to be relevant to their times. Chapter 7 picks up this question and related issues when discussing the role of the citizen therapist.

In sum, if we can find a way to integrate commitment and community into our emerging emphasis on interpersonal connection, we potentially have a new cultural ideal: the relational self. It's an antidote to the poison of the consumer self. In terms of psychotherapy, the relational self means that no problem can be treated as if it is contained only within the individual client. Healing occurs within a web of interconnected, committed bonds, personal and communal. As I once heard family therapist and Ojibway tribe healer Sam Gurnoe say, "Outside of a culture, a community, and a spirituality, you can treat but you cannot heal" (personal communication, 1995).

2 THE CRAFT OF ETHICAL CONSULTATION IN THERAPY

I recall a seminar where a senior colleague and trainer described a case that had haunted her.[1] She was seeing a married couple for sexual problems that were exacerbated by significant psychological problems in both spouses (I don't recall the details) and a highly conflicted relationship marked by periods of escalation and then withdrawal. Among their many problems was the reason they were seeing my colleague: They were not able to have sexual intercourse, and the wife's individual therapist thought that a skilled sex therapist might be helpful. This was just a challenging clinical presentation for my colleague until she asked why they wanted to work on their sexual relationship now. They responded, "We want to have a baby." When the therapist asked why a baby now, they replied, "We think a child would bring us together."

Imagine you are the therapist. How would you feel if this couple told you they wanted to work on getting pregnant? What would you worry about, if anything, and how would you communicate your concerns to them in a supportive way?

---

[1]The case examples in this chapter have been modified to disguise the identities of the clients involved and to protect their confidentiality.

https://doi.org/10.1037/0000263-003
The Ethical Lives of Clients: Transcending Self-Interest in Psychotherapy, by W. J. Doherty

Like my colleague, you would probably feel dismayed. You would be worried for them if they were to have a child right now. You would be worried for the child born into their family. You would foresee a train wreck if they succeeded in their goal. You would know you have to raise your concerns in a therapeutic way.

My colleague reported that she did her best to help them understand the challenges they would face in bringing a child into their lives right now. She began by asking them what they thought it would be like to take care of a baby, given the personal and marital difficulties they were facing. They waved her off: "We know it would be hard, but it's something we would deal with together, and that would bring us closer. Plus, we've always planned to have a child, and now seems like the time." The therapist went through a list of specific burdens of taking care of an infant, and again, they said they were confident they could manage.

So far, we are in the realm of clients taking personal risks that their therapist is more concerned about than they are. It's the stuff of regular clinical practice, as when a client says she wants to go back to her old boyfriend, and the therapist sees more potential harm than the client does. Our job is to look around corners that our clients may not be focusing on and pose questions and concerns in a way that respects their autonomy. My colleague did all of this and was troubled when her clients kept responding, in effect, "We hear you, and we see the risks differently. Now let's move on with the sex therapy."

What's the ethical issue here? It is not the couple's decision to take on a challenge that their therapist considered unwise; that's a matter of self-determination by two adults who were capable of making their own choices. The ethical issue is the potential harm to a baby who would come into their lives when they were struggling just to take care of themselves. (Recall the care/harm dimension of moral foundations theory described in Chapter 1 and our working definition of the ethical realm in therapy: client behavior that has consequences for the welfare of others.) The not-yet-conceived child was an ethical stakeholder in the couple's decision making. The therapist understood this, and, as a mother of young children herself, she felt it deeply.

The quandary for the therapist was that she didn't know how to bring up her ethical qualms. She had exhausted the traditional clinical path of inviting her clients to consider how having a child would affect their well-being and then firmly but gently challenging their perceptions of the risks. Now she could think of just two alternatives: say nothing further because it's the clients' decision, not hers, or flat out tell them that they should not try to have a child now because they couldn't take care of it. Neither seemed right: the first one because it felt like walking away from concern for the child and the second one because telling clients what to do was not good therapy practice.

As I listened to my colleague, I had several thoughts. First, if this highly skilled therapist, who never seemed at a loss for the right thing to say, was paralyzed about approaching a client's ethical issues, I was confident that the great majority of therapists would feel the same way in this and other ethically fraught situations. Second, at the level of the craft or skills of ethical consultation, my colleague could come up with only two unsatisfying extremes: Keep quiet, or tell the clients what to do. It was A or Z and nothing in between—abandon the ethical field or take it over. Third, I saw a middle path for this case, not because I was the smallest therapist in the room but because I had consciously developed some skills for addressing ethical issues in therapy. I had options other than A or Z. In other words, these situations are hard but not paralyzing if you have a repertoire for addressing them.

I've used this case in workshops for therapists in the following way: I present the case and ask what the ethical issue is. Participants have no trouble seeing that the ethical issue is about the needs of the baby and the potential harm involved. I explain how the therapist addressed the risks of harm to the couple, the couple's response, and the therapist's dilemma about how to proceed. I then invite workshop participants to write down, word for word, how they would introduce the ethical dimension to the couple. I explicitly tell them to focus on the ethical issue of care/harm for the baby and not on trying additional ways to show the couple that it would not be good for them to have a child. In other words, I ask them to focus on the ethical claims of the child and not the self-interest of the couple, which, although clinically important, had already been thoroughly explored.

Astonished is how I feel every time three fourths of workshop participants only come up with additional ways to help the couple understand that having a child would be bad for them personally. Examples include "Let's walk through what a night and early morning are with a newborn," and "Are you familiar with what research shows about the effects of a first child on a marriage?" I acknowledge that those are useful questions but not in the ethical domain. I keep steering participants back to the question of how to address the interests of the child. At first, I thought the problem was in my directions for the exercise, and then over time, as I made my directions clearer and more explicit, I concluded that many therapists are not able to think in terms of addressing third-party claims when talking with clients. It's as if I were asking them to switch to a foreign language: How would you ask a question in Greek?

Keep in mind that by this point in the workshop, I had given a definition of the ethical realm in therapy, I had critiqued therapy's exclusive focus on self-interest, I had presented moral foundations theory, and I had described several cases, including the story of Bruce recounted in the Introduction. And the setup for this case emphasized that the ethical issue concerned the child. After a half dozen participant responses that focused exclusively on helping the couple see what would be harmful for them—to which in role-playing one of the spouses, I responded with reassurance that we could handle the stress—I finally heard responses focusing on the child as a stakeholder in the decision. Some of these responses were cautious and even clumsy, such as turning the session into an explanation of infant and child development in hopes that the couple would spontaneously realize that they are not able to meet the child's needs. Eventually, a handful of responses directly and respectfully addressed the needs of the child in light of the struggles the couple is currently experiencing. The bottom line here is that the skills of ethical consultation are more difficult than they appear to be, given the training of therapists to avoid the ethical realm in therapy.

After working with workshop participants about what they say to the couple, I end with the words for the couple that I offered to my colleague: "I want to ask you about something you've no doubt thought about. Given the personal and relationship struggles you've been having, what do you think it would it be like for a baby who came into your lives right now?" This is not therapeutic rocket science; it just puts the ethical issue on the table for the couple to ponder. The therapist is not silent on the ethical front, does not tell them what to do, and does not dance around the issue but instead invites a conversation about how the client's decision might affect the well-being of someone for whom they would be responsible.

My therapist colleague took in my input and said that, indeed, she could have asked that question and followed up with some gentle challenges if the couple seemed unaware of the challenges the baby would face. However it turned out, she would have a path into an ethically grounded conversation. Instead, she said ruefully that she had found herself doing the slowest sex therapy of her career, and the couple eventually dropped out before restoring their sexual relationship.

Next, I describe the skills involved in ethical consultation with clients. I go back and forth between the terms *craft* and *skill*, with some preference

EXHIBIT 2.1. Craft Skills in Ethical Consultation

The Basic Skills: LEAP (Listen, Explore, Affirm, Perspective)

- Listen for the client's ethical language and moral emotions.
- Explore moral intuitions, emotions, beliefs, and meanings.
- Affirm the client's ethical sensibilities and sense of agency.
- Perspective:
    - Frame both sides of a dilemma.
    - Encourage the client to emphasize a moral intuition that seems muted.
    - Invite the client to take the role of someone affected by the issue.

Advanced Skill: Challenge

- Pivot from LEAP interactions.
- Forecast that you are about to say something challenging.
- Affirm the client's autonomy.
- Express worry about the effects of the client's actions on someone else.
- Switch back to expressing empathy.
- Suggest that the client may be temporarily blinded by one set of feelings.
- Directly contradict the client's minimization of the effects on others.
- End most challenges by again affirming the client's autonomy.

for the former because it connotes a body of technique honed over time in a community of practice. The model is outlined in Exhibit 2.1.

THE LEAP-C MODEL OF ETHICAL CONSULTATION

In most ways, discussing the ethical concerns of clients is no different from talking about other issues in their lives. The skills are not exotic. The challenge is to be able to listen for ethical dilemmas and engage them as such, using moral and ethical language as appropriate. This section first addresses the basic craft that is usually enough when the client brings an ethical dilemma to the therapy. These basic skills are framed in the acronym LEAP: listen, explore, affirm, and offer perspective. The subsequent section describes the more advanced skill of challenge (C), when the client does not perceive an ethical dilemma and the therapist decides to bring it up. The LEAP-C skills are generally used in a linear fashion: first, listen, then explore and affirm according to what you are hearing from the client, and only then offer a perspective if that would be useful. (As I note, sometimes the client resolves the dilemma without the therapist offering an explicit perspective.) Using ethical challenges would only be appropriate in certain situations (described later) and after the LEAP skills have been brought into play. To be clear, however, I am not offering a prescription that these skills must always be used in sequence; the complexities of clinical conversations allow space for therapist judgment about what to say when.

Listen for Clients' Ethical Language and Moral Emotions

Engaged listening is the quintessential skill of good therapy. In the context of ethical consultation, it refers to the ability to hear ethical intuitions and emotions when clients raise them, without immediately translating ethical language into more comfortable and familiar clinical language. One of my clients, an older woman who has a middle-aged son with multiple sclerosis in a nursing home, was torn between wanting to visit him every day—a trip that takes her several hours—and her retired husband's expectation that she be home with him. In terms of clinical language, one way to frame her situation is her internal conflict between making her own decisions to prioritize her time (in this case, to visit her son) and her husband's demands that she be available to him. This challenge no doubt has roots in her earlier life, their marriage, larger cultural issues related to gender, and much more, depending on your clinical model. As she talked and I listened and explored her situation, the immediate ethical dimension became clear: She felt an obligation to support her son and check on his care, while at the same time, as a traditional wife, she felt a duty to take care of and please her husband. Although, of course, I worked with the clinical issues in this case, I also let her know that I understood her ethical dilemma, which in moral foundations theory related to the domains of care and fairness—namely, does care for her son contradict her fairness to her husband?

I explored this client's dilemma not in academic language but in terms of the burden she felt every day as she left for the nursing home because she felt she had to check in on her fragile son, knowing that she was disappointing her husband, who wanted her home with him. She was caught between two obligations and feeling awful whatever she did. The ethical considerations deepened our work because they reflected a core part of how she was experiencing the problem. We also explored her sense of how her husband was coping with the decline of their son's health, with the possibility that her visiting every day might stir up his feelings of guilt for not seeing his son very often. She soon concluded that her son's need for regular contact and support was greater than her husband's desire that she be home. She expressed that conclusion to her husband with sensitivity, and he ceased complaining. She felt lighter in the world after finding her ethical moorings. In terms of the LEAP-C skills, I mostly used listening and exploring. I can't recall whether I explicitly affirmed her moral commitments to her son and her husband, but I am confident that she felt my support. I did not need to use the perspective skill because she got to a resolution by exploring the issues with me. If she had remained paralyzed, I might have offered this kind of perspective statement: "As I listen to you, I find myself thinking about who is the most vulnerable person in your life right now: your son or your husband. If your husband were seriously ill and in need of home care, that might tilt you toward staying more with him because your son has providers to look after him. Right now, though, your son seems to be in more need of support. Your husband would like you to be around more, and that's important to consider, but your son is in a tough spot right now." I would be looking for the client's nonverbal responses as I offered this perspective, and I would end by tossing the ball back to her: "Those are some thoughts I have at the moment." And I would let her carry the ball from there.

An everyday example that nearly every therapist has encountered is a married client framing a decision about divorce not only in terms of pain in the marriage (which would be a reason to leave) but also in terms of marriage vows and commitment. As mentioned, I was trained in the 1970s to ignore the ethical part of the client's dilemma and focus only on the client's sense of what would be better for the self—to stay and perhaps try to make things better for the self or leave and seeking happiness elsewhere. But research has shown that ethical concerns beyond self-interest (particularly about commitment and children) are commonplace among people considering divorce (National Divorce Decision-Making Project, 2015). The question is whether therapists give these concerns appropriate space in therapy by taking them seriously as specifically ethical concerns that clients are processing in terms of their moral integrity and not just in terms of the costs and benefits to themselves. Most of our clients don't separate the psychological and the moral, even if we are trained to do so.

Explore Moral Intuitions, Emotions, Beliefs, and Meanings

After we learn to tune our therapeutic radar to ethical dilemmas when clients raise them, the next step is exploring what is going on for the client. In most ways, the craft here is not different from exploring clients' experience in any other area of their lives, such as relationship concerns, feelings of anxiety or loneliness, and so forth. However, given the individualist bent of traditional psychotherapy and therapists' sensitivity about shaming clients, it can be tempting to simply note a client's ethical dilemma or emotions and not follow up to understand it more fully. When a client expresses strong guilt or shame about a past action (e.g., "I feed bad that I hurt/cheated somebody"), the therapist may choose to normalize the action immediately (e.g., "You were young," "You had bad role modeling"). The goal is to protect the client from feeling bad about the self. Ironically, the same therapist would not hesitate to encourage the client to go into more depth about any other painful feeling. We are still dealing with Freud's legacy of moral emotions as inauthentic expressions of societal norms residing in the superego (Jones, 1966; Zaretsky, 2005).

Therapists often have just a few seconds to decide whether and how to follow up on something clients share that seems outside of the scope of therapy. Take medical issues that clients bring up. Until I worked in medical settings and got comfortable with medical issues, I often did not follow up right away when clients mentioned a medical condition. I didn't say, for example, "Tell me more about that," "How is it affecting your life?" or "How are others responding to you?" A medical doctor was handling that part of their life, I told myself, and I thought I needed additional expertise to have an extended conversation about the role, say, of diabetes in a client's life. I came to see that I was truncating the therapy by holding back from exploring the impact of health problems because I was defining my role too narrowly. (See McDaniel et al., 2014, for an alternative way of working with clients who have medical problems.) Clients get the message and keep medical issues out of the therapy office when they sense the therapist is not interested. The same can be true with ethical issues.

I recall an intake with a couple when the husband clarified that although he had been married once and they had one daughter, he also had a young adult son from an earlier, nonmarried relationship. He then said, "I still feel guilt over not having a relationship with my son." He paused and added parenthetically, "I don't know if guilt is healthy" and ended with "But that's part of my motivation to make this marriage work for my daughter." When I heard him express self-doubt about the feeling of guilt, I noted to myself that he had been well socialized by years of therapy to wonder whether guilt is an inauthentic or unhealthy emotion. It's a way of "shoulding" ourselves, which we used to say in 1970s encounter groups was a way of "shooting" ourselves.

I followed up with an exploratory question: "You say you feel guilt about your relationship with your son. Could you say more about how you've been a father to him and what you regret?" The client went on to say that he had entirely exited his son's life after the breakup and deeply regretted that decision but that in the last year, he had reconnected with this son and was now trying to do right by him. This was part of a new narrative he was writing for his life, one in which he tried his best to follow through on his commitments. My acknowledgment that I had heard him, followed by a simple exploratory question, opened up this dimension of his life for our work.

The ethical consultation skill of exploring, then, generally begins with a question that takes seriously the moral experience of the client and goes from there. What is the client's meaning regarding the experience? Who are the other players in the narrative? If it's a current dilemma, as in the previous example of the older mother, what feelings and beliefs are connected to each choice on the table?

Lest this seem straightforward for therapists, I want to point out the temptation to take clients off their own ethical hook by referring only to the conditions and forces that led them to a decision they now regret. With the man who abandoned his son, of course, it's entirely appropriate for the therapist to help him see the context of his choice: Abandoned by his father, hooked on drugs, in a bad relationship, and with little money to spare, he was set up to walk away from his son when his partner ended the relationship. (There is literature showing how overdetermined these choices are for many low-income fathers; Edin & Nelson, 2013.) Understanding the context of decisions can help clients develop a more complex narrative for pivotal moments in their lives and not collapse into self-loathing. We therapists are good at helping clients move away from simplistic self-blame. However, our training and therapy models, for the most part, do not help us be as good at helping clients accept self-responsibility and moral agency and own realistic guilt about actions that have harmed others.

One more example of the problem that this book addresses: I watched a training video of a famous therapist interviewing a couple in which the husband was taking responsibility for the years in which he avoided dealing with his wife's emotional distance by going to a local bar and attracting the attention of women by telling sad tales of how he couldn't get through to his wife even though he loved her dearly. He had convinced himself that this behavior was okay because it was a safety valve for his frustrations, and he had never had a sexual affair with any of these women. Now he was willing to say that he was being irresponsible and putting his marriage at risk. (In terms of moral foundations theory, his moral intuition was in the domain of fairness to his wife.) He spoke with a sense of perspective on himself, offering self-effacing humor about his well-rehearsed act and with what seemed to be an appropriate level of guilt or self-reproach.

When I watched that video segment, I thought, "This is beautiful. He is not just admitting 'mistakes' based on being in a difficult marriage but also saying that what he did was self-gratifying at the expense of his marriage." Then I was dismayed when the therapist responded (not a direct quote but the essence of the therapist's comment), "But you were lonely and couldn't reach your wife who was walled off from you. That's why you sought attention elsewhere. It was all part of the marital dance." The husband was not buying it. After listening to the therapist repeat various versions of how the marital interaction pattern led to his actions, he politely repeated that his wife had not made him show off for other women and play the emotionally available but lonely husband. The therapist responded again with another "but" and dug into how his family of origin issues had set him up to respond this way to a distancing wife. The husband let it go, and the therapist moved on.

For me, this session showed how even a gifted therapist could have a failure of moral imagination. The therapist's model had sophisticated ways to explain the sources of dysfunctional marital behavior but seemed not to have a place for moral agency. So rather than explore the client's newfound sense of conscience and how this could help the marriage, the therapist kept reinterpreting his experience in language that had no place for ethical self-knowledge or accountability. I concluded that this was not just a random mistake—we all miss key opportunities in sessions—but a blind spot in the therapist's model itself.

What would ethical exploration look like in this case? Questions such as the following are examples:

- "What were you telling yourself when you first began to go to the bars?"
- "Looking back, how did you justify it to yourself?"
- "When did you begin to have doubts about whether what you were doing was right?"
- "What specifically seemed wrong?" (If he said it was unfair to his wife, I would ask how it was unfair.)
- "Because you were getting a lot of rewards out of this, how did you come to sacrifice those rewards and turn back to your marriage?"
- "Did you get input from anyone else along the way?"

Exploration like this would create a richer therapy experience instead of a partial experience where the client has to stay within the confines of a clinical model and clinical language stripped bare of ethical dimensions central to the human experience.

Affirm the Client's Ethical Sensibilities and Sense of Agency

Along with sensitive listening and deep exploration, affirmation is another pillar of the practice of psychotherapy. We affirm clients when they have important insights or try out constructive new behavior. We appreciate them for taking risks inside and outside the therapy office. It's no different in the ethical realm, provided we are attuned to this dimension of the human experience. The barhopping husband in the prior example would have benefited from an affirmation when he came clean on what he had been doing—for example, "What you're saying now is really important. It sounds like you've been doing some major soul searching."

In general, ethical affirmations are simple interventions, not complex ones. They have to come spontaneously in the moment and from the therapist's heart, or otherwise, they will sound patronizing ("Good husband!"). Sometimes an affirmation comes at the end of an exploration that leads the client to confront something not accepted before: "I appreciate how hard you've worked in this conversation to be honest with yourself and about what you've done. This is not easy."

Sometimes an affirmation can be quite brief, as when the mother in a family arrived a couple of minutes late for a family therapy session and said, "I'm sorry I am late. I was taking care of my mother. As you know, she's dying and in hospice. [Pause and a sigh] She was not the best mother in the world, but I feel an obligation to be there for her as she's dying." My response was, "Of course you do," a simple affirmation of her sense of moral obligation. Now comes another example of how therapists can miss moments like this and worse. After I told this story the next week in a graduate class, a student approached me after class with her own experience in therapy as her own mother was dying. She had been seeing a prominent therapist and used almost identical words to those of my client. Her therapist responded with a question regarding the student's mother: "What is she to you now?" The question was delivered in a challenging tone. My student said she felt a paralyzing chill go through her body, with part of her appalled at what the therapist had just said and part of her doubting her own ethical sensibilities regarding her mother.

To be clear, I understand that exploring a client's relationship to a dying parent is grist for therapy (including a soft version of the question of how the client feels about the parent now). And perhaps my student recalled the incident incorrectly. But it does fit a pattern of therapists not knowing what to do with clients when they use ethical language—and then turning it into a challenge. Here's a thought experiment: What would seem more sophisticated as reported in a case consultation—my brief affirmation ("Of course you do") or this therapist seizing the moment to challenge her client to reconsider her dysfunctional attachment to her mother? For context, let's not forget that clients spend a lot of their time in therapy discussing the negative aspects of their relationships with mothers and other family members—and relatively less time on the history of positive aspects of these relationships, let alone their enduring commitment to these people, which can lead a therapist to question why the client would make sacrifices for this family member (Schwartz, 2005).

Offer Perspective

The bulk of ethical consultation in therapy stays with the LEA skills: listen, explore, and affirm. Generally, clients come to a meaning or decision that works for them. They don't need the therapist to offer a perspective on the ethical issue or dilemma. The father who felt guilty about abandoning his son did not need me to offer a perspective on the ethical dimensions of fathering. If my sex therapist colleague's questions had generated enough reflection on the needs of the baby, the couple may have decided to use contraception until they were in a better place to become parents. I had a client who was torn about whether to tell his difficult twin brother about a new medical diagnosis that could be genetically related. My client decided to do so after I asked this question while exploring the situation: "If your brother were in the same situation with a new diagnosis, what would you want him to do?" The client responded, "Tell me, of course. That's why I have to do the same for him." I asked why he was now so clear, given his fears about being vulnerable with his brother. His response still leaves me emotional: "Because he's the only person on this earth with my genes. I have to tell him so he can take care of himself." The client came to his own conclusion based on my exploring the dilemma and asking a key question (I call it the Golden Rule question).

To reemphasize a point: In general, my approach to ethical consultation is "less is more." Listening, affirming, exploring—these are usually enough. In other cases, when the client is stuck on making meaning of past behavior or making a decision about current or future behavior in the ethical domain, it can be useful to offer a perspective. Next are three specific ways to implement the craft of sharing ethical perspectives with clients.

Framing Both Sides of a Dilemma

As mentioned, a common ethical dilemma therapists see with adults is whether to divorce or stay in a marriage. Most clients express concerns about their own happiness and well-being if they stay in the marriage, given their level of emotional distress. And most clients with children express worry about the effects of divorce on their children. This is a classic ethical dilemma: a personal happiness stake and potential downsides for others who are dependent on us. As mentioned, I used to collapse the dilemma into one pole: What would be the better outcome for the self because, presumably, children will be fine if their parents do what is best for themselves? I later learned to honor and frame both sides of the dilemma without weighing in on which side I thought the client should lean toward—for example, "I can appreciate how hard this decision is for you right now. You're deeply unhappy in your marriage and can't see a way to make it better, and you're also worried about how a divorce would affect your kids when they seem to be doing okay right now." This kind of framing best uses words that the client has already expressed in the session, giving both sides of the dilemma equal weight. The goal is to help the client clarify the elements of the dilemma. Chapter 3 goes into more depth about ethical consultation on the divorce decision.

Encouraging the Client to Emphasize a Moral Intuition That Seems Muted

A client is struggling with a decision on honoring her mother's request to stay in her own home versus moving her to an assisted living facility. The bind is that she is worried about her mother's ability to live independently, though she also wants to respect her mother's strong desire to stay at home. This is a clear ethical dilemma, with potential harm both ways and no clear better path at the moment. As the client describes the situation, the therapist notices that she is focusing on the interpersonal challenge of going against her mother and dealing with that guilt and the reaction of her mother. In other words, the client is emphasizing just one moral intuition: respect for her mother's authority over her own life (the authority/subversion foundation in moral foundations theory). To bring more balance to the client's thinking about the dilemma, the therapist can say, "I hear your concern about disrespecting your mom's wishes to live independently by forcing her into assisted living. You want to do right by her. [Wait for the client to acknowledge that she has been heard.] Of course, there is the other side that I know is on your mind: the potential harm to her if she stays in her house." In this way, the therapist brings a both/and perspective to the client's deliberations by bringing to the fore something that the client feels and believes but is not prominent in her discernment at the moment—in this case, the care/harm dimension.

Inviting the Client to Take the Role of Someone Affected by the Issue

It's tempting for all of us to emphasize harm to ourselves but downplay harm to someone else who is affected by our behavior. This kind of ethical blind spot is particularly likely when we are at odds with someone such as an ex-spouse with whom we share children. It's easy for parents to downplay the effects on their children of words and actions regarding the ex-spouse. For example, for emotional self-protection, a parent might ask a child to be the bearer of negative news to the other parent, as in asking the child to report that there will be a schedule change that will inconvenience the other parent. Here is how I address this with parents: "I hear how upsetting it is to deal with your ex directly. I get why you ask your daughter to speak for you. I'd like to also invite you to think about how your daughter feels when she carries messages that upset her mom." Here I am doing two things that are important in ethical consultation: acknowledging the client's experience and the reasons for their actions and posing a question that invites the client to take the perspective of someone affected by their behavior. When this is done skillfully, clients rarely react negatively; they are usually aware of the potential effects that the therapist is inviting them to consider. When a basic invitation like this does not register with the client (such as when a parent claims the child is not bothered by bearing bad news), an advanced skill might be needed: how to challenge a client on ethical grounds.

BEYOND LEAP: ETHICAL CHALLENGE

Therapists who hear about ethical consultation sometimes imagine that it's about telling clients that they are doing something wrong and they should stop doing it! That indeed would be poor therapy. As I've stressed, most ethical consultation occurs in low-intensity, nonconfrontational exchanges where the emphasis is on "consultation"—helping someone sort through their thoughts and feelings, with the therapist occasionally directly sharing a perspective on the client's dilemma. However, there are situations when a good consultant in any area (financial, career, medical, and so forth) may have to move into the territory of challenging a client about something.

Of course, skills in challenging clients are part of the standard toolbox of therapists. Imagine a scenario in which a woman client is thinking of returning to an abusive boyfriend. The therapist explores her rationale and the emotions and experiences underneath that rationale. The therapist probably hopes that this kind of exploration will lead the client to decide to stay out of this harmful relationship. If that does not "work," many therapists will increase the intensity of their intervention, perhaps by directly challenging the client's belief that her boyfriend has changed because he is now being sweet when he calls her or because he says he has stopped drinking (but has not gone to treatment or AA). The therapist might express worry for the client's safety. All of this can be done with a lot of support and affirmation. But it's within the traditional individualist approach to therapy, where the therapist is there to promote the personal interests of the client—for example, extricating herself from an abusive relationship. It's not ethical consultation as I define it in this book.

The difference with ethical challenges is that it's not mainly about the needs of the client but about how the client is affecting someone else. This is more paradigm rattling for therapists than challenging a client about self-defeating behavior. And, of course, it's riskier than other ethical consultation skills we've covered because the client might feel unfairly pushed or judged. What are some situations where ethical challenges might be useful despite the risks? Here are four scenarios:

- when the client has an ethical blind spot about harm to another: in the prior example, a parent who does not see the damage from putting a child in the middle of a conflict with the other parent;

- when the client is acting inconsistently with core personal values—for example, a married person who professes the value of marital fidelity but justifies an emotional affair as harmless,

- when harm to another is imminent—for example, a divorcing parent is about to reveal the other parent's affair to a young child, along with a moral condemnation; and

- when exploration and perspective regarding these issues have not helped the client understand the ethical stakes involved.

I begin with how not to challenge in the ethical realm. It's important to enter the domain of challenges with intentionality and not when triggered by the client's blind spot or actions. I've heard the following mistakes reported in supervision and case consultations. The first is making pronouncements about one's values or "biases." (Some therapists who do not like to talk in terms of ethical values use the latter term.) I think of a young therapist who, when a single mother said that she did not want her child's father involved in their lives, responded, "I want to say up front that I believe that fathers are very important to their children." Pronouncements like this put the therapist and client in antagonistic positions. The therapist may feel better, but the client probably does not.

The second mistake is to lecture the client about professional wisdom and research findings in hopes that the client will yield to the therapist's "higher" knowledge. This is pronouncement making in a more professional-sounding form. Of course, research can be brought up in therapy, but the mistake is to present it in a didactic manner to get the client to change their thinking when the client has not responded to exploratory interventions. I have heard therapists describe their lengthy presentation on attachment theory when talking with a parent who is not doing right by a child. Clients know when they are being lectured to, and they often respond with, "Yes, but."

The third common mistake is to advocate for others while not connecting with the client's emotional stress. This stance is especially tempting when therapists are triggered by a parent's actions with their children. I once viewed the video of a session where the therapist, presenting a teaching case at a national workshop, repeatedly confronted a biological father in a step-family about the urgency of his taking more leadership with his daughter. (He had mostly abdicated responsibility to his new wife, and his daughter appeared to be acting out to get his attention.) The father kept repeating that he was under immense pressure (his first wife had died, stepfamily life was hard, and his work pressures were immense). The therapist did not acknowledge his emotional distress and kept starting her responses with variations of "But your daughter needs you right now." This part of the session ended with the therapist lecturing the father on male privilege in today's society and the father shutting down. To repeat, this was not a bad day at the office; we've all blown it with clients. This was a teaching video presented by a leading therapist showing what the therapist considered good work.

What are some skilled ways to challenge clients on ethical grounds? I lay them out in brief form here and return to some of them in later chapters. Again, I want to stress that these are not used frequently in ethical consultation and that it's important for a therapist to be intentional and skillful when it's necessary to challenge clients about the effects of their behavior on others.

- **Pivoting** from LEAP interactions by asking permission to offer a different perspective than the client's ("I have a different take on how your wife might be feeling about your affair. Is it okay if I share it?").

- **Forecasting** that you are about to say something challenging ("I have a challenge for you to consider about how you are viewing this situation").

Both pivoting and forecasting prepare the client for what is to come. It's important to look for a verbal or nonverbal agreement for you to proceed.

- **Affirming the client's autonomy** before offering a challenge ("The decision on this is yours, not mine or anyone else's, and I'm not living in your shoes").

- **Expressing worry** about the effects of the client's actions on someone else. Recall my comments to Bruce, the father who was thinking of walking out his children's lives, about how this could affect them permanently (see the Introduction).

- **Switching back to expressing empathy** for the client's distress and affirmation of the client's good intentions ("I know you are swimming as fast as you can right now and that it sounds like I am encouraging you to do the impossible").

• **Suggesting that the client may be temporarily blinded** by one set of feelings (e.g., anger at an ex-spouse) and not accessing another set of feelings (e.g., concern about the children).

• **Directly contradicting** the client's minimization of the effects on others. A recently separated client had just learned that her husband was seeing another woman. Even though she had agreed not to say negative things about her husband to the children, she called me on the phone to say our no-negativity agreement was over. She was going to tell their emotionally vulnerable 11-year-old son that his father was a morally corrupt adulterer because he deserved to know the truth about his father. After calling on the history of our therapy work and what I hoped was her sense that I cared about her, I said, "I know you are terribly hurt right now. I also know that saying this to your son will hurt him terribly, both now and in the future." She softened and said that she was tired of painting her husband in rose-colored glasses to the children. I affirmed that it was time to stop doing this but that she did not have to paint him at all. She pulled back from her decision and agreed to talk more about this in our next session.

• **Ending most challenges by again affirming the client's autonomy** in making their own life choices ("I appreciate how you've listened to my concerns, and I want to say again that I don't get a vote in what you decide. We can do good work together no matter how you decide to move forward").

Challenges in the ethical realm can put stress on the therapist–client relationship. They have to be done with calm, care, and compassion, not out of a reactive desire to rescue someone. In most cases, the therapeutic relationship is strengthened because the therapist is taking a risk from a place of concern for both the client and others in the client's life.

To finish this chapter on the theme of craft, one of the difficulties for therapists in the ethical realm is that we have lacked an explicit set of skills to develop, discuss, debate, refine, and pass on skills to new therapists. I don't pretend that I have the final word on the craft of ethical consultation. What I offer is open for consideration by my colleagues. This has to be better than the current state of affairs in the field where either we avoid important ethical issues in the lives of our clients, or we make things up on our own and then keep quiet about it with colleagues.

PART **II** COMMON ETHICAL
DILEMMAS IN
CLIENTS' LIVES

3 KEEPING OR ENDING COMMITMENTS

A life without interpersonal commitments is a life untethered. Notice that I did not say a life without "relationships," which can be fleeting. Commitment comes with obligations and an open timeline. It often involves sacrificing immediate needs. The person I am permanently committed to knows I'm invested in their well-being and makes life plans accordingly. However, if I'm in an intimate relationship that does not involve a permanent commitment, all I owe the other person is a respectful goodbye if I'm ready to move on. The same for most friendships: I don't owe friends years of hard work (and maybe therapy) to maintain a relationship that has become hurtful for an extended time. In other words, committed relationships have an ethical dimension that simply being in a relationship does not.

In the world of therapy, we have barely begun to take the ethics of commitment seriously as we work with our clients. To make this point more charitably: The therapy literature is rarely explicit about the moral dimension of commitment in how we work with clients in relationship difficulty. (There is scholarly work outside of therapy on interpersonal commitment—for example, Stanley, 2005, and Tran et al., 2019.) In this chapter, I focus on how therapists can support (and how they sometimes inadvertently undermine) commitment in

https://doi.org/10.1037/0000263-004
The Ethical Lives of Clients: Transcending Self-Interest in Psychotherapy, by W. J. Doherty

two important relationships: marriage (by which I mean a lifelong, intimate relationship) and adult relationships with their parents (particularly as the parents become frail).

THERAPY AND MARITAL COMMITMENT

Shortly after I finished writing *Soul Searching* in 1995, the therapy blind spot with the ethics of commitment came home to me in the form of stories I received from married people who were close to me. In telling their stories, which they gave me permission to do, I am aware that it's possible that they misunderstood their therapists or did not recall the details correctly. However, they are all credible people to me, and their stories fit a pattern I have heard from many clients over the years about their experiences in therapy. This pattern includes stories from fellow therapists about their experience as clients. In other words, although I can't vouch for the accuracy of any particular story, I can be confident in the overall trend.

Monica, a relative of mine, called from another city to say that she was stunned when Rob, her husband of 18 years, announced that he was having an affair with her best friend and wanted an "open marriage."[1] When a shocked Monica refused to consider this alteration in their marriage, Rob bolted from the house and was found the next day wandering in a nearby wood. After 2 weeks in a psychiatric hospital for acute psychotic depression, he was released to outpatient treatment. Although during his hospitalization, he claimed that he wanted a divorce, his therapist urged him not to make any major decisions until he was feeling better. Meanwhile, Monica was beside herself with grief, fear, and anger. She had two young children to care for, a demanding job, and a chronic illness diagnosed 12 months before this crisis. Indeed, Rob had never been able to cope with her diagnosis or with his job loss 6 months after that.

Clearly, this couple had been through huge stresses in the past year, including a relocation to a different city where they had no support systems in place. Rob was acting in a completely uncharacteristic way for a former straight-arrow man with strong religious and moral values. Monica was now

---

[1]This case example is from "Bad Couples Therapy: How to Avoid Doing It," by W. J. Doherty, 2002a, *Psychotherapy Networker*, (November/December), pp. 26–33 (https://dohertyrelationshipinstitute.com/wp-content/uploads/2019/11/Bad_Couples_Therapy.pdf). Copyright 2002 by The Psychotherapy Networker, Inc. Adapted with permission. The case examples in this chapter have been modified to disguise the identities of the clients involved and to protect their confidentiality.

depressed, agitated, and confused. She sought out recommendations to find the best psychotherapist available in her city. He turned out to be a highly regarded clinical psychologist. Rob was continuing in individual out-patient psychotherapy while living alone in an apartment. He still wanted a divorce.

As Monica recounted the story, her therapist, after two sessions of assessment and crisis intervention, suggested that she pursue the divorce that Rob said he wanted. She resisted, pointing out that this was a long-term marriage with young children and that she was hoping that the real Rob would reemerge from his midlife crisis. She suspected that the affair with her friend would be short lived (which it was). She was angry and terribly hurt, she said, but determined not to give up on an 18-year marriage after 1 month of hell. The therapist, according to Monica, interpreted her resistance to "moving on with her life" as stemming from her inability to "grieve" the end of her marriage. He then connected this inability to grieve to the loss of her father when Monica was a small child; Monica's difficulty in letting go of a failed marriage stemmed from unfinished mourning from the death of a parent.

Fortunately, Monica had the strength to fire the therapist. Not many clients would be able to do that, especially in the face of such expert pathologizing of their moral commitment. I was able to get her and Rob to a good marital therapist who saw them through their crisis and onward to a recovered and ultimately healthier marriage.

In another case close to home for me, Jessie, a friend of my family, emailed me upset when her new counselor, whom she was seeing for depression and complaints about her marriage of less than a year, suggested that she consider a trial separation from her husband because an unhappy (but not highly conflicted) marriage was keeping her from feeling better. Jessie recounted the exchange: When she told her counselor that she was committed to her husband, the therapist kept repeating that she may not be happy again if she stayed in this marriage and that a "break" might help her. Upset with this counselor, Jessie turned to her priest, who also stunned her by suggesting that if her marriage problems were causing her depression, he could help her get an annulment, given the newness of the marriage. As with Monica, Jessie turned to me to ask whether this kind of undermining intervention was common in the field—and what she should do next.

In another example, the anxious wife of a verbally abusive husband who was not dealing well with his Parkinson's disease reported that she was told at the end of the first therapy session in her HMO, which offered only brief therapy, that her husband would never change and that she would either have to live with the abuse or get out.[2] She was grievously offended that this young therapist was so cavalier about her commitment to a man she had loved for 40 years and who was now infirm with Parkinson's disease. She came to me to find a way to end the verbal abuse while salvaging her marriage. When I invited her husband to join us, he turned out to be more flexible than the other therapist had imagined. He, too, was committed to his marriage, and he needed his wife immensely. That was the leverage, along with a change in medications, for him to start treating her better.

One of my students experienced serious postpartum depressions after the births of her two children. She told me that both of the therapists she had seen at different times challenged her about why she stayed married to a husband who did not understand her needs. (Her husband was befuddled by his wife's moods and sometimes became impatient with her, but he was not, according to my student, a mean-spirited man.) In the first session, one therapist said in a challenging tone of voice, "I can't believe you are still married." Although it's fully possible that my student invited these responses by potent criticisms of her husband, it's the job of a therapist to hold the presenting sentiments of a depressed, postpartum client with a degree of caution before giving advice about ending a marriage. However, as Schwartz (2005) observed, because of our empathic engagement, therapists are "powerfully drawn to our patient's point of view in their assessment of others" (p. 276).

A final illustration involves a friend who went to a well-regarded therapist for his depression. After a number of months, the therapist requested that his wife come to a session. The following week after the conjoint session, the therapist recommended that, on the basis of what she had observed and heard from the client, he consider divorcing his wife. My friend responded emphatically that divorce was not on the table for him and that he loved his wife and was committed to her. The therapist persisted, maintaining that his marriage problems were complicating his depression. My friend pushed back even harder: "There is not an ounce of interest in my body for divorcing my wife." The therapist's final words were, "I'm just asking you to think about it." As in the other stories, my friend contacted me for help in understanding what had just happened, wondering whether this was standard care in the field. In this case, part of his confusion was that he felt he had

---

[2]This case example is from "Bad Couples Therapy: How to Avoid Doing It," by W. J. Doherty, 2002a, *Psychotherapy Networker*, (November/December), pp. 26–33 (https://dohertyrelationshipinstitute.com/wp-content/uploads/2019/11/Bad_Couples_Therapy.pdf). Copyright 2002 by The Psychotherapy Networker, Inc. Adapted with permission.

received excellent treatment from a therapist he had sought out because of her strong reputation. How could a therapist who seemed so thoughtful and skilled in treating his depression be so clueless and undermining when it came to his commitment to his marriage?

WHY MANY THERAPISTS APPROACH MARITAL COMMITMENT THIS WAY

These illustrations should not be dismissed as examples of random bad therapy or incompetent therapists—or just the biased recollections of the clients. (As I said, although no doubt clients sometimes misinterpret their therapists, when similar stories come up repeatedly, including from colleagues as clients, they cannot be dismissed.) In my view, these stories reveal the challenge for many therapists of how to think about and address clients' life commitments in situations when those committed relationships are sources of pain and distress. It's not that therapists deliberately undermine marriages; the rub comes when the marriage seems to be harming their client or keeping them from achieving their therapeutic goals. As I have repeatedly argued, when we lack a way to think about ethical issues in everyday life, we fall back on the mainstream cultural priority of individual self-interest. We challenge clients to privilege their immediate self-interest over relational commitments. This looks like neutrality, but it's a heavily value-laden stance, one the therapist is usually not conscious of holding in an individualistic culture.

I was not immune to this way of working as a young therapist. I learned to treat the divorce decision with what I thought was neutrality. I remember working with Mary Ann, a 35-year-old woman in an unhappy marriage who wanted individual help to decide whether to keep working to change her marriage or end it.[3] She and her husband had two small children. This was the height of the divorce boom in the 1970s, and a number of her friends had recently left their husbands. Mary Ann felt stifled in a bland relationship with a man who didn't connect with her emotionally in the way she wanted and who expected her to do the lion's share of the parenting and housework, along with her part-time job. Sound familiar as a marital complaint? As I sat

---

[3]This case example is from "Couples on the Brink: Stopping the Marriage-Go-Round," by W. J. Doherty, 2006, *Psychotherapy Networker*, (March/April), pp. 30–39 (https://dohertyrelationshipinstitute.com/wp-content/uploads/2019/11/Couples_On_the_Brink_Networker.pdf). Copyright 2006 by The Psychotherapy Networker, Inc. Adapted with permission.

with her, I realized that I'd never been taught how to work with someone on the brink of divorce. My training in marriage therapy started with the assumption that both parties wanted to stay together, at least for the time being. My training in individual therapy had taught me that my job was to help my clients clarify their feelings, needs, and goals and then make their own decisions without my values and viewpoints getting in the way.

So, I did a kind of rational-choice consultation with Mary Ann, helping her clarify what she'd gain or lose personally from her decision. "How would your life improve from leaving your marriage," I asked, and "What might it cost you to leave?" I asked the same about staying: "What are the pluses and minuses of remaining in the marriage?" (I was studying statistics at the time and even imagined a two-by-two contingency table!) When she worried aloud about the effects of a divorce on her kids, I responded, "The kids will be fine if you're happy with your decision." Mary Ann ultimately decided to file for divorce and start a new life.

Even at the time, I felt odd about treating this client's dilemma as if it were a decision that only affected her. And I felt sad that another not-so-bad marriage was biting the dust. Not that I'd have admitted this to a supervisor or peer because a hallmark of a good therapist in my circles was to be cool about the rash of divorces we were seeing among our clients and peers. No one wanted to come across as a moralistic marriage saver. Divorce was a hard-won right and a legally supported, no-fault personal choice. At this point in the early 1980s, Putnam (2020) observed that "expressive individualism framed marriage as a limited liability contract dissolvable with a 'no fault divorce'—'expressive divorce'" (p. 152). The common wisdom was that a therapist should not get too involved beyond clarifying the options and supporting the client's autonomy.

Looking back, I'm struck by my naiveté about what's involved in leaving a marriage, especially one with children, and my innocence about my lack of influence on the outcome. Like most people facing this decision, Mary Ann was caught in a morass of ambivalent feelings and values. (Harris et al., 2017, documented the volatile ups and downs of divorce decision making.) She'd made a lifelong commitment to her husband and now was considering withdrawing it. She wondered whether her expectations for this husband, or any husband, were realistic. She hadn't done much psychological work on herself and didn't have an idea of what good marriage therapy might accomplish. She worried about her economic future, and she was deeply concerned about the effect of a divorce on her children, who'd lose their daily connection to their father, take a financial hit, and face a series of substantial life changes. She also believed that her parents and friends would be shocked and upset with her if she left the marriage.

Mary Ann's journey toward her decision was, like most people's, highly unstable and marked by ambivalence (National Divorce Decision-Making Project, 2015; Vaughn, 1990). But despite this instability and the high stakes, I treated her as if she were thinking of changing jobs from Walmart to Target: What does each company offer you, and what would be the downside of staying or switching jobs? And, by the way, you owe nothing to your current employer as you make this decision. Maybe her choice of divorce was the best one, and maybe she would have made the same choice regardless of how I'd worked with her. But she deserved a complex therapy to match the complexity of her dilemma, not an oversimplified, "neutral" therapy that failed to engage both sides of her ethical dilemma. Her husband, children, and future grandchildren also deserved better from me. As the novelist Pat Conroy (1978) famously wrote, "Each divorce is the death of a small civilization."

As therapists, we are midwives for relational deaths and rebirths, the shattering and rebuilding of committed intimate relationships that are at the heart of human experience. But you won't find much training, writing, or even conversation among therapists about how we handle these moments in therapy. The result is that we're each left to make things up on our own, mostly using the implicit ethical norms embedded in our culture and profession.

ADULTS' COMMITMENT TO THEIR PARENTS

Riding in an elevator once in Singapore, I saw a sign for one of the floors of the government center labeled something like "Parent Court." When I inquired, I learned that it was a place where parents who felt neglected by their adult children could seek the help of the court to enforce filial obligations. I knew I wasn't in Kansas anymore! In the United States and similar Western countries, adult children have no legal obligations to care for their parents (just as the parents have no legal obligations to their children when they turn age 18). Adult familial relationships are voluntary in the ethical realm, not the legal one.

The field of psychotherapy has been hard on parents from the beginning, seeing them as primary sources of the pathologies in their offspring. Whether it's toilet training in traditional Freudian theory or inadequate attachment bonds and authoritarian or permissive discipline in contemporary models, there are plenty of parent deficiencies to sort through with clients in therapy. However, I suspect that the working assumption among therapists was that you could work to recover from poor parenting in the past while still having a relationship with your parents in the present. That began to change in the 1980s with the rise of cultural interest in "the dysfunctional family," including intrafamilial sexual abuse and codependency on problematic parents and other family members (Bass & Davis, 1988). Parents were not just toxic influences from the past; they were continuing to harm their adult offspring in the present. What's more, they could be a threat to their grandchildren.

From the mid-1980s through at least the mid-1990s, many therapists joined the recovered memories movement in the field, believing without evidence, for example, in the near pervasiveness of multiple personality disorder brought on by intrafamilial sexual abuse (Acocella, 1999). I recall case consultations where therapists, again without evidence, said that 90% of women with bulimia had a history of incest in their families. The next wave was about the since-discredited claim of widespread satanic ritual abuse of babies and children. The upshot was a wave of therapist-encouraged cutoffs from parents and often from other family members who did not accept the claim of that abuse. Parents would receive "goodbye" letters, crafted with the encouragement of therapists, from their adult children, especially their daughters who were more apt than their sons to be in psychotherapy. Our field got caught up in a huge wave of cultural negativity about family life (Wylie, 1993).

Eventually, there was a cultural pushback, highlighted by a *New Yorker* article and subsequent book by investigative journalist Lawrence Wright (1994) on satanic cult accusations and an acclaimed PBS *Frontline* episode, "Divided Memories" (Bikel, 1995), which featured a high-profile therapy clinic where nearly all clients were encouraged to achieve the goal of "detachment" by cutting off from their parents and, in some cases, from their spouses and even their children while they recovered their sense of self. In these and other cases around the country, the therapists involved were proud of their work and had a theoretical model behind it (if no research data). After successful lawsuits ensued, therapists quietly abandoned their practice of suggesting family abuse via recovered memories, and they stopped taking as accurate the notion of large numbers of dead babies as a result of satanic cult abuse.

But the idea of a therapeutic cutoff from parents (and siblings who ally with the parents) had been loosed in the field and continues in practice and books by therapists for the lay public, such as Campbell's (2019) *But It's Your Family . . .: Cutting Ties With Toxic Family Members and Loving Yourself in the Aftermath*. That author described in detail how she came to cut off all contact with her pathological father and mother, and she urged the same for her readers after they evaluated whether the criteria she offered fit their parents.

In the mid-1990s, as my own children were entering college, I gave a presentation to a group of college counselors that included interns and staff. The topic was the value of seeing college students as members of families instead of just as emancipated individuals. I will never forget an exchange with a junior staff therapist who asked, "Aren't there times when the student's family is so toxic, not only in the past but also still now, that it's best that the student break off a relationship with them?" I replied that I had seen some tragic cases where the past abuse was not only denied but also continued with intensity and that in those cases, it can be useful for a young person to take a time-out from connecting with family. Then I thought to ask, "I'm curious. For what percentage of your caseload do you believe a family cutoff would be called for?" I froze in my chair when he said, "Maybe 40%." The chill I felt was that I was soon to launch my oldest child to college—what if he developed emotional problems and saw this therapist? No one present offered a counterview, and we moved on after I mumbled something about this not being my experience. In retrospect, I wish I had challenged him about how he came to his perspective. It was a failure of nerve on my part that I vowed never to repeat.

I have heard many clients report encouragement by therapists to end relationships with parents and other family members, and I've seen this in my extended family. These days, whenever I hear about a definitive cutoff from family, I ask whether there is a therapist in the picture. To be clear, I believe that these therapists want to help their clients avoid unnecessary emotional pain by encouraging them to exit relationships that continue to cause this pain. It's not that therapists hate families or that there are never situations that call for a strategic time away from abusive family members (in my mind, always with the hope for later reconciliation). Rather, these therapeutic interventions reflect a cultural orientation where all relationships are transactional—what is the benefit I am gaining versus the cost to my well-being? If the relative psychological cost of maintaining a family relationship is too high, the healthy thing to do is to end it. I later return to the case of Laura, whose story opened this book on the note of adult commitment to a difficult parent. Here I just note that Laura told me that she had several therapist friends who encouraged her to "ditch" her mother.

Missing here are two ideas: first, that parent–child bonds are not psychologically disposable—they go on until the death of the parent and beyond—and second, that there is an ethical dimension to the parent–child (and other family) relationship. A permanent cutoff means that adult children have no moral obligation to respond to their parents' current needs and the eventual frailty and end of life. These two levels—psychological and ethical—go together. Like it or not, we are emotionally tethered to our parents and they to their adult children. Therapists come and go, but not parents. As I've heard the psychologist Mary Pipher (2008) say, "Nobody calls out for their therapist on their deathbed" (p. 2).

I don't have a one-size-fits-all formula for obligations to parents, especially when the parents are in need of support and help. There are so many factors, including the history of the relationship. Obligation to a parent who abandoned you at birth and has now reentered your life wanting support will look different from obligation to a parent who has shown consistent care and support over the years. How much to be involved personally, with openness and vulnerability, with a frail or dying parent will depend on how much emotional safety there is in the relationship. Then there is the complex issue of what forms of help are, well, helpful. As asked earlier in this book, when is taking a parent home to one's own house the best decision for all concerned versus placing the parent in a care facility? Culture comes into play here: In some cultures, an out-of-home placement is seen as an act of cruelty, while in others, is it considered loving when done at the right time.

My main point here is that the job of the therapist is to help the client navigate these difficult waters, discerning the interests of the self, parent, one's spouse and children, and others. Moral foundation theory can help to sensitize us to competing ethical intuitions: Care/harm, fairness/reciprocity, and respect for authority seem particularly relevant here. Good ethical consultation does not mean that the therapist has the answers but that the therapist honors the client's commitment to parents in light of all the other factors involved.

THE CRAFT OF ETHICAL CONSULTATION ABOUT COMMITMENT

I use the LEAP-C (listen, explore, affirm, offer perspective, challenge) skills to demonstrate strategies for ethical consultation when commitment to a marriage or a parent relationship is on the table—that is, when a client is struggling about staying in a marriage or about cutting off or withdrawing support from a parent in need.

Listen

Listen for the ethical part of the client's decision making. For marriage, it might be a dilemma over personal happiness versus the original commitment or the needs of the children. For adults with their parents, it might come out in the form of the client's guilt, sometimes accompanied with resentment, over not doing enough for one's parent. As with all forms of listening in ethical consultation, it's important to give a full hearing to both sides of the dilemma and to how the client is expressing a number of moral intuitions in light of their life experience and their culture, including intuitions such as authority and loyalty that do not come readily to mind for a Western therapist. In Laura's situation with her challenging, soon-to-be-frail mother, I listened carefully to her ambivalent feelings and thoughts: on the one hand, self-protective ones for herself in the face of current and future burdens (the current one focused on her mother's criticisms, and the future one added more caregiving) and, on the other hand, a sense that it would be wrong to cut off her mother. Her friends were listening mainly to the self-protective side of her ambivalence. Laura said she came to me for therapy because she believed I would also listen to the other side.

Explore

The nuances emerge during exploration. For parent dilemmas, these include the quality of the relationship now and in the past, the possibility of manipulation versus genuine need, the availability of other caregivers such as siblings, and the resources of the client to help the parent in light of other obligations. Often a decision will emerge from this exploration, one that the client can live with in terms of resolving the tension between personal needs and responsibility for parents.

For Laura, the exploration revealed the details underlying her sense that she could not just walk away from her mother: It didn't seem right as the only child of a widowed parent. But she also lived with an emotional burden of listening to her mother's weekly phone monologues about how others don't treat her fairly, including her daughter. Her mother also offered critiques of Laura's mothering (those hurt the most). I especially paid attention to how the client responded to her mother on these calls, uncovering how passive and annoyed she would become but not set limits. This exploration opened up possibilities for her to remain regularly in her mother's life while building healthier boundaries.

In terms of marital commitment, the following is a series of exploratory questions that I developed for a specialized approach to couples work called discernment counseling, where at least one spouse is considering ending the marriage (Doherty & Harris, 2017):

- What has happened to your marriage that has gotten you to the point where you are considering divorce? Notice that this is not framed as "What are the problems?" or "Why are you unhappy?" but in terms of the marriage being a major part of the client's life that is now under question.

- What have you or your spouse done to try to repair the relationship—to fix the problems before you got to the point where divorce is on the table? This question carries the assumption that marital commitment is worth an effort to find a way to maintain—the relationship deserves repair attempts if it's broken.

- What role, if any, do your children play in your decision making about the future of your marriage? This delicately crafted question brings the needs of the children into the conversation in a way that gives the client space to respond in a variety of ways.

- What were the best of times in your relationship since the time you met—the times you had the most connection and joy? This question brings clients back to what they used to love about their spouse and what led to their original commitment.

The point behind questions like these is to show that exploring ethical dilemmas over commitment can involve more than "tell me about both sides of your struggle." There are lots of nuances and often more than two stakeholders—for example, third parties such as children who will be affected by the decision. Laura, for example, weighed the effect of a parental cutoff on her children, who would grow up without contact with the grandmother.

Affirm

Affirming involves acknowledging and supporting the client's ethical commitments. In Laura's case, I explicitly affirmed her moral sense that she should not take her therapist friend's advice to "dump" her mother like a bad boyfriend. I used words like these: "I appreciate that you want to do right by your mother even though she's a difficult mother. It's not easy, but you've decided it's important that you stay in her life, especially at this time when she's pretty much alone." Laura sat up straighter in her chair and said, "Right. That's the path I have chosen. Now I want to figure out how to do this and keep my sanity."

Affirmations on divorce decisions are trickier because of the inherent volatility involved for many clients in coming to a conclusion. When clients bring up their ethical concerns, say, about their marriage vows or the children, I affirm them without suggesting that those concerns are determinative—they don't necessarily mean staying in the marriage. It's just that commitment has an important role in the decision. In contrast to how I used to dismiss these concerns, I've learned to simply acknowledge and accept them with language such as "I appreciate that you are taking seriously your original commitment to your marriage; leaving is not something you take lightly," or "I hear your concerns about the children, and I'm glad you are taking these concerns seriously. There is a lot at stake all around." By the way, many older clients with adult children and grandchildren are concerned about hurting these stakeholders. I affirm that concern as well. And, of course, I affirm the client's right to think about their pain and harm to self from staying in a bad marriage and their concerns that a highly conflicted marriage can also be harmful to the children. That's why it's an ethical dilemma: There are legitimate needs and claims in tension.

Perspective

As mentioned, it's often not necessary to share one's perspective on an ethical dilemma because clients sort out how to proceed with the help of the listening, exploring, and affirming skills. In situations when commitment is in play, however, clients can often benefit from the therapist's perspective on how to have a healthy, satisfying life while maintaining commitments to others, such as a difficult spouse or a burdensome parent. Self-sacrifice for the sake of ethical commitments can be difficult to sustain and, in some cases, may not be healthy or wise (as with an abusive spouse who will not seek help).

In the case of Laura, I shared a perspective this way:

ME: I hear you on your desire to be a supportive daughter to your mother—saying goodbye to her is not an option for you. Now let's talk about how you can support her in a way that's healthy for you. The current situation is not working: You feel burdened by her weekly calls, stressed for a day beforehand, and upset for a day or more afterward. You go through the week with negative thoughts about her and then feel guilty for being so negative. Do I have that right?

LAURA: Yes, exactly.

ME: So, your bind is that you don't feel like a good daughter when you are in touch with her, and you would not feel like a good daughter if you abandon her. [Notice that I used explicitly ethical language— "good daughter"—because the client had been using that kind of language. I did not substitute nonethical language such as "responsive" or "measuring up."]

LAURA: Oh, my, yes!

ME:　　So, let's think together about two things: What might be going on for your mother that she acts this way and how you can learn a healthier way to interact with her. Right now, it doesn't seem as if you have good boundaries with her on the calls—you let her go on and on, and when she criticizes you as a mother, you've said you defend yourself and feel angry at her. My idea is that we would work to find a way for you to have healthy boundaries with your mother on these calls so that you feel you are there for her and protecting yourself at the same time. And by the way, it's not healthy for your mother when she treats you poorly. So, a better-boundaried relationship would be good for both of you.

Here, I was offering a perspective on how Laura could take care of herself and her mother at the same time. Over the course of our work, she did find helpful ways to listen to her mother's complaints about her life while at the same time setting firm limits when her mother started to offer personal criticism of Laura's mothering. All of this was standard therapy work on my part. The point of emphasis for present purposes is that I framed this, in part, as ethical work, a way to resolve a moral challenge for the client who had wondered whether it was unhealthy of her not to walk away from her mother as others, including her therapist friends, had advised her.

In terms of offering perspective on divorce decisions, a key is to honor both sides of the ethical dilemma in two main ways:

- **Normalize the dilemma.** It's hard to know the right decision when dealing with ongoing personal suffering and hopelessness in a marriage, along with struggles about abandoning one's commitment and putting one's children at risk. And most people go up and down in their decision making.

- **Share concerns.** When a client seems to be making an impulsive decision to divorce (say, right after learning of a spouse's affair), the therapist can share some general wisdom about the value of slowing down in making a lifetime decision. I like to use the phrase of a wise collaborative divorce lawyer: "Divorce is never an emergency; it takes months to play out." A separation can be an emergency decision when there is threat and risk, but deciding to divorce rarely has to be done immediately and in emotional turmoil. Another example of perspective is when a client seems to be downplaying a future consequence of a divorce. I recall a married man who thought that his adult children would readily accept his lover (because she was such a great person) if he ended the marriage to be with her. I offered an alternative perspective so that he could be more realistic in his decision making: the likelihood of resentment from his children, at least for some time. A final example was a client in a volatile marriage who said that he could just stay away from his wife until the last child left home in 6 years. I offered that I've seen this work sometimes for couples who already have a lot of distance and little conflict, but I wasn't sure it would be feasible in his more engaged, high-conflict relationship, especially if it was his unilateral decision to stay married but be functionally single.

Challenge

To discuss challenges in intergenerational commitments, I switch to parent to child commitment because it's more commonly needed there. Recall my discussion in the Introduction about Bruce, who was about to move away and abandon his children after his wife kicked him out of the house. When I asked him the exploratory questions of how he thought leaving his children would affect them, he replied, "I'm sure it will bother them for a while, but they'll get over it before long." Given the urgency of the risk (Bruce had come to what he said was a final session to wrap up our work before he left town), I decided to immediately challenge him with these blunt words: "I don't think so. Walking out of their lives will affect them for a long time, even permanently." Bruce soberly replied, "I know you're right." I asked why he thought what I said was right. "They will feel hurt and not understand why this happened. You know, I left my daughter in California the same way, and I think about how it affected her. I don't want to do that again, but I don't know if I can go back to that house and see my wife, not in the state that I'm in." Bruce and I were now in accord that he wanted to keep his commitment to his kids. Our work now was to figure out how to do this while maintaining his fragile emotional equilibrium.

Ethical challenges require a caring relationship so that they don't come across as judgmental. I recall a divorced father who learned that his 7-year-old son was calling his new stepfather "Dad." My client felt terribly hurt and replaced. I empathized with his feelings. Then he told me that he had told his son that day that if he ever heard that he was calling his stepfather "Dad," he would never see the child again. I was shocked and worried for the child, but I held on to the craft of ethical consultation by first connecting with my client:

ME: Joe, I know you are in a lot of pain about your divorce and scared to death about losing your kids' love and affection. And I know that you would never intentionally harm your children. [*Slight pause*] I also have to tell you that what you said to Bobby probably hurt and wounded him and left him fearing that he could lose you. You are the only father he has, and he should not have to live with the fear that if he slips and calls someone "Dad," he will lose you forever.

JOE: [*Looking worried*] Do you think he could feel that way? I just wanted to get through to him about me being the only one he calls Dad.

ME: I'm really worried for him right now. That was a big threat you made to him.

JOE: I can see it now. I was beside myself upset, and I took it out on him. What do I do now?

We went on to discuss how he could repair what he had done, beginning with contacting his son right after our session. We went over the words he could use to apologize and offer reassurance that his commitment was forever and not contingent on something his son would say.

Most therapists would be with me in cases of parent commitment to young children: Ethical challenges can be appropriate there. When it comes to marital commitment, many therapists take a neutral stance on whether clients divorce and would be reluctant to go beyond sharing perspectives for the client to accept or not (Wall et al., 1999). My view is that while there can be good reasons to let go of a marital commitment, it's a weighty ethical decision because it affects the welfare of at least one other person who made life decisions based on an expectation of continued commitment, and usually, there are additional stakeholders such as children and extended family members. Therefore, I am willing to challenge clients when I believe they are not including concern for other stakeholders in their decision making. Keep in mind that challenge generally only comes after using the other skills of listening, exploring, affirming, and offering perspective. Here are some examples:

- **Challenging a client to seek couples therapy.** "I'm concerned that you are leaving your marriage without seeing whether it could be become healthy again through good couples therapy."

- **Challenging a client to let a spouse know the marriage is on the brink.** "I realize you don't think your spouse can change. Maybe so, maybe not. What I want to challenge you about is not signaling to her that you are so unhappy that you are considering divorce. It seems to me that she is owed a chance to see whether she wants to make changes that might preserve the marriage. She's flying blind now."

- **Challenging a client about ending a good-enough marriage when the client is depressed or in a personal crisis.** This challenge can take two forms: appealing to self-interest ("I'm worried that you will do something that you will regret when you are in a better emotional place") and appealing to the interests of others ("This decision is going to affect a whole lot of people, such as your kids, and I'm worried that it's hard for you to fully consider those consequences when you are feeling the way you do. You could look back with regret about the fallout").

I end this chapter's discussion of ethical commitment with words I wrote in *Soul Searching*:

> Our therapy caseloads are like Shakespearean dramas suffused with moral passion and moral dilemmas. But we have been trained to see Romeo and Juliet only as star-struck, tragic lovers, while failing to notice that the moral fabric of parental commitment was torn when their families rejected them because of who they loved. We focus on the murder of Hamlet's father and Hamlet's own existential crisis, rather than on how Hamlet's mother abandoned her grieving son. Commitment to loved ones, and betrayal of that commitment, are central moral themes in the human drama played out in psychotherapy every day. (Doherty, 1995, p. 46)

4 HAVING AFFAIRS

Cheryl was married for 17 years and had two teenage children.[1] About a year before our consultation, which was requested by her therapist, who felt stuck with the case, she'd begun an affair with a man she knew professionally and was now paralyzed about making a decision of whether to stay in her marriage or move to another town to be with her lover. Her job took her out of town about once a month, when she and her lover got together for great sex and conversation. Her affair partner started divorce proceedings with his wife and was pressing Cheryl for a commitment to leave her marriage and be with him. As we began our conversation, she said she was experiencing a "churning dilemma."

I asked about her marriage. She said that her husband was a good man—kind, loving, and supportive—but that the marriage lacked passion for her.

---

[1]This case example is from "Couples on the Brink: Stopping the Marriage-Go-Round," by W. J. Doherty, 2006, *Psychotherapy Networker*, (March/April), pp. 30–39 (https://dohertyrelationshipinstitute.com/wp-content/uploads/2019/11/Couples_ On_the_Brink_Networker.pdf). Copyright 2006 by The Psychotherapy Networker, Inc. Adapted with permission. All case examples in this chapter have been modified to disguise the identities of the clients involved and to protect their confidentiality.

https://doi.org/10.1037/0000263-005
The Ethical Lives of Clients: Transcending Self-Interest in Psychotherapy, by W. J. Doherty

She'd felt emotionally empty for a number of years, and their sexual relationship had become infrequent and unexciting. She believed they were doing a good job of raising their children, and her husband had supported her career decisions. In fact, he was so supportive and constructive that she was confident that he would not leave her or be mean-spirited if she told him about the affair.

But, she said, she deserved more out of life and marriage than she felt she could get from her husband. Fear of hurting her children was keeping her from leaving. They'd be devastated, she thought, and their lives would be turned upside down, especially if she moved away to be with her lover. After years of passively accepting a loving but passionless marriage, she felt that she'd come alive after being kissed by a man who'd been her friend and later her lover.

As I listened to Cheryl tell her story, I concluded that hers was not an abusive or destructive marriage but rather a supportive and companionate one that seemed to be meeting many of the needs of the children, her husband, and even Cheryl. If she'd told me her husband was violent, addicted, or chronically irresponsible, I'd have thought about her situation differently because sometimes starting an affair is a wake-up call to seriously consider getting out of a destructive marriage. Either way, though, continuing an affair creates damage to the spouse who is being lied to and betrayed and at risk of a sexually transmitted disease. So, there were multiple ethical issues at stake in my ethical consultation—the marital commitment, the secret affair, and the potential consequences for a number of stakeholders. In moral foundations theory terms, the issues involved care/harm and fairness/cheating.

I saw Cheryl as operating out of what I call a "consumer" approach to marriage—focusing on what benefits she wasn't receiving from her husband and not on what she was failing to put into the marriage. And I believed there would be harm to her children and husband if she were to end her marriage at this point. As I listened to her, I reflected on the research demonstrating that the children who experience the most harm from divorce are those whose parents have relatively harmonious marriages, even though not especially happy or intimate (Booth & Amato, 2001).

Cheryl struck me as a caring, sensitive person, but she spoke about her desires as if they were constitutional rights, such as freedom of speech, and her emotional needs as if they were biological facts, such as needing vitamin C to avoid scurvy. Our culture teaches us that we're all entitled to an exciting marriage and great sex life; if we don't get them, we feel deprived and permitted to go elsewhere to meet our needs. What used to be seen as a weakness of the flesh has mutated into an entitlement of the psyche. Cheryl clearly sensed that her secret affair and accompanying deception were wrong in a moral sense, but like many people in satisfying affairs, she found ways to rationalize her choices. My point is that in 21st-century Western culture, consumer entitlement to a fulfilled life is a compelling reason to enter and remain in situations we know are ethically compromising.

Although it lurks inside most married people in our mainstream culture, the consumer attitude usually doesn't become apparent until we come face to face with our disappointments about our marriage and our mate. Then we start to ask ourselves, "Is this marriage meeting my needs?" and "Am I getting enough back for what I'm putting into this marriage?" In Cheryl's case, she'd told herself for years that she'd "settled" for a second-class marriage for the sake of the kids.

During the first 20 minutes of the interview, I focused on helping Cheryl explore the implications of the affair and leaving her husband for her well-being. Using the metaphor of the affair as a vacation paradise, an exotic island where no one can actually live permanently, I tried to undermine the fantasy of a blissful new love relationship that would never encounter the decline in passion that nearly all long-term relationships experience. I also presented a scenario in which she could see rebuilding her marriage as a positive option for herself instead of a sellout of her core personal needs. Because she'd eventually end up on the "mainland" anyway—in a long-term relationship, with its daily responsibilities and challenges—why not figure out how to have a satisfying marriage with her current husband. She said she liked that option but was doubtful that it was possible.

Toward the end of this first part of our conversation, Cheryl explicitly said that she'd consciously chosen the affair and was no longer "a good girl." I know how I'd have handled this comment during the 1970s: I'd have encouraged her to challenge the way society or religion or her rigid conscience were defining her as no longer "good." I'd have supported her heroic efforts to break out of the mold of following other people's expectations for her.

Instead, I let her remark pass without comment or follow-up. Given the urgency of her decision making and the high stakes, I moved the conversation to the realm of interpersonal ethics—how her behavior and decisions might affect others in her life—rather than focusing on her claims to authenticity and rebellion from conventional standards. Future therapy could return to the theme of her being a good or bad girl to see whether she could integrate these parts of her identity, but for now, I wanted to shift her gaze outward rather than inward.

In a pivotal part of the interview, I summarized and validated the aspect of her decision associated with her self-interest and then asked her to reflect on the consequences of her leaving. The following are excerpts from the transcript.

"Okay. So, there are two parts of this," I said. "One part is where you might have your best chance for personal happiness—to live in this new relationship so that the next part of your life may give you more joy. And then the other part of the decision concerns the consequences to different people."

"Yes, I know, I know," she responded.

"So, let's talk about that part of it."

"The consequences?" Cheryl asked.

"And maybe we can put your personal happiness and the consequences for others back together at some point. But, for now, how do you think a divorce would affect your children?"

This question represents a core part of ethical consultation: asking about how the client's actions might affect the welfare of someone else. I've never had pushback from this kind of question, delivered in a plain, matter-of-fact manner. Why not? Nearly all clients have been asking themselves this question, even if therapists sometimes tremble about putting it forward. "How would this affect someone else?" is the quintessential ethical question; it's also a thoroughly human question because we all know we impact one another as interdependent social creatures.

Cheryl didn't even let me finish the question: "Oh, the consequences would be devastating," she said. We explored her sense of those consequences, especially for her children, and I affirmed my concern as well. The next key moment in the interview followed my statement that it's possible for couples who work at it to "have the kind of energy and passion that's truly fulfilling—not the same as that of a new relationship but the kind of passion that, after 10 years or 15 years or 20 years, you say, 'Wow, this is good.'" "Yeah, see, I can't believe that," Cheryl replied. "It's unbelievable to me that that's possible." "In your marriage?" I queried. "In my marriage, right," she said. "So, keep talking, so you can tell me more how to do that."

At this point, I had an okay to lay out a path in which Cheryl would end the affair definitively and tell her husband that their marriage had been in grave danger and that she'd had an affair. A little later, when she challenged the idea of telling her husband about the affair, I said that I don't have any firm rules about this sort of thing but that my sense was that this level of honesty would give both of them their best chance to make some major changes. He would understand the jeopardy his marriage had been in and perhaps be motivated by that knowledge.

During the remainder of the interview, I tried to undermine Cheryl's sense of fatalism that her husband could not change. I did this by challenging her passivity in the marriage and her unrealistic beliefs that, somehow, her husband should respond with grand, dramatic, romantic actions to her ambiguous, half-hearted gestures toward improving their relationship. Near the end of the session, I repeated the theme that Cheryl, at some point in her life, would have to do the hard work of maintaining an intimate marriage, even if she left her current marriage for her lover. "So, I might as well do it in my marriage because we've got history in the marriage, and it would be hurting so many people for me to leave," she responded. "That's for you do decide," I said. "That's for me to decide, yeah," she agreed. "But that sure makes sense to me," I concluded. Notice that I reaffirmed her autonomy in this important decision. I also gently supported the direction in which she appeared to be leaning because my position was no doubt quite clear to her anyway I then encouraged her to work through the decision with her therapist.

Cheryl ultimately took back her marriage from her affair. She ended that relationship and started working on her relationship with her husband—not without sadness, though, about letting go of the dream of a new relationship that would be a permanent love affair. Then an emotional crisis with one of her children helped to rivet her attention back to her family. She regained her marital commitment when she understood what was at stake: a long-term marriage, a husband who loved her, children who depended on that marriage, and a community of people affected by the marriage. She'd been focusing on what she was not getting from her marriage, what she was entitled to get, how her husband's flaws had created her dissatisfaction, and how she'd be happier with a new model of husband. In the end, she came to see that she held citizenship papers in her marriage and only a tourist visa in her affair. When I followed up with her therapist a decade later, I learned that both she and her husband had made changes, and the marriage is doing well.

THE CLINICAL AND ETHICAL COMPLEXITIES OF AFFAIRS

In addition to divorce decisions, affairs may be the main ethical issue that therapists encounter in the everyday practice of adult psychotherapy. There is extensive therapy literature on how to help couples recover from an affair (e.g., Baucom et al., 2011; Hertlein et al., 2005) and lots of lay literature on how to recover from a spouse's affair (e.g., Gordon et al., 2018; Spring, 2013) but little on how to counsel a married (or similarly committed) person who is in the midst of an affair or reflecting on a past affair. Filling this gap, at least in terms of the ethical dimensions of affairs, is the goal of this chapter.

It's clear that most clients think of their affairs in ethical terms, even if therapists prefer to think just clinically. Even as U.S. society has become more accepting of sexual behaviors previously disapproved of—such as non-married sex and same-sex relations—the level of disapproval for extramarital sex remains high, higher than in the relatively permissive 1970s (Hemez, 2016). The term "cheating" remains common, even as terms such as "living in sin" (for cohabitation) have disappeared. I think the reason is that, for most people, extramarital sex in the form of secret affairs is seen as an unacceptable violation of an expectation that the partners will be sexually faithful. It's the unilateral cancellation of a core part of the marital agreement. Even couples who practice polyamory have agreements about how, when, and with whom they will have outside sexual relations with—in other words, they're not engaging in secret cheating (Haritaworn & Klesse, 2006).

The ethical ramifications of affairs can involve sexual actions, lying and deception, and sometimes betrayal through the involvement of someone connected to the spouse. An example of all three dimensions is a case where a husband had a secret, long-term affair with his wife's good friend and daily coworker. And then there are ethical dimensions involving children, putting the stability of their family at risk because of an affair. If the affair partner is married with children, the ethical ramifications multiply. And then there are emotional affairs.

Emotional Affairs

During my training, we didn't have a clear concept of marriage-threatening relationships that were not sexual. In those more gender-separate days, we debated whether it was possible for men and women to have close friendships that did not move into the sexual domain. (In the "heteronormative" world I lived in, we did not consider the question of nonsexual friendships for gay people.) Nowadays, there is lay and professional awareness that married people can get into close relationships that undermine their primary relationship without being explicitly sexual (Moller & Vossler, 2015). In many cases, the people involved tell themselves that it's not cheating on their spouse. But the effect on the spouse and the marriage can be similar when the other relationship becomes emotionally more salient and rewarding than the primary relationship—or when the other person becomes a competitor to the spouse in other ways (such as via comparisons or secret sharing), usually without the spouse knowing it.

In addition to entering a relationship that can threaten marital commitment, the main ethical dimension of emotional affairs comes in the form of lies and secrecy about the existence or importance of the other relationship.

For example, a husband, when describing his day at work, omits the long cappuccino break with his coworker. Or a wife, when listing which colleagues are going on a business trip, leaves off the name of someone she is looking forward to spending time with. Texts arriving at home from that coworker or friend are reported as coming from a relative. For a time, the spouse is in the dark about the other relationship, and when they begin to express worries, their mate denies or minimizes. Thus, deception becomes part of the fabric of the marriage in a way that ethically compromises the spouse having the emotional affair.

Ignoring the Ethical Dimension of Affairs

It's possible for therapists to see themselves as doing good therapy while disregarding the impact of a client's affair on others. In the mid-1990s, there was public discussion of the secret affair of Woody Allen with his long-term partner Mia Farrow's 19-year-old daughter, which eventually led to a divorce from Mia and a marriage to his stepdaughter, Soon-Yi Previn. A major issue in the custody trial over the younger children was Allen's fitness as a parent. According to a *New York Times* journalist who covered the proceedings, it did not go well for the therapists who were called as expert witnesses (Marks, 1993). When pressed by an attorney about whether they thought it was wrong for someone to have a secret sexual relationship with a spouse's daughter, the therapist witnesses would not give an ethical opinion. In language that reminded me of witnesses during the Watergate hearings of the 1970s, they used language such as "error in judgment" and "a mistake under the circumstances." One therapist, someone I personally know and admire, even explained the unusual sexual arrangement as a reflection of the postmodern family. At that point, the exasperated judge sternly cut him off with these words:

> I find it extraordinary the words that therapists use who come here, and they can say "bad judgment" or "lack of judgment." But isn't there something stronger? You went through the "postmodern structure of the family" and types of relationships. We're not at the point of sleeping with our children's sisters. What does it mean? (Marks, 1993, p. 3)

Here is my take on this embarrassing scene. These therapists, who were invited to testify because they were experts, were in a bind. They likely saw ethical language and moral judgement as inconsistent with the role of the therapist. Thus, if they had used moral/ethical language in responding to questions, they would be acting unprofessionally. In other words, if a true therapist is value neutral, then using value-laden language about someone's behavior means you are not a good therapist, let along an expert one. The incredulous judge, along with many journalists who wrote about the trial, spoke for ordinary people who don't refrain from moral considerations when reflecting on human behavior.

Several years later, I had a chance to comment publicly on the Allen case. I was doing a New York public radio interview in which the interviewer mentioned the Allen case and asked whether I had ethical qualms that I would address if I were Allen's therapist. I responded that I would raise the issue and would press it even if he dismissed my concerns about the impact of his actions on his stepdaughter, his wife, and the rest of their children. The interviewer was with me all the way and said he would be appalled if a therapist saw it as not their role to invite a client in Allen's shoes to examine the moral dimension of his actions. It turned out that the first caller to the radio show was also appalled—by my stance! She said she was a psychoanalyst who was fully committed to not judging clients but instead to helping them explore the psychological dynamics of their life choices. The interviewer took her on, asking her whether she would remain silent about the train wreck that Allen's behavior was risking. She replied that challenging a client about their impact on others was not her job and that doing so was bad therapy. She then added that if Allen's step-daughter had been under age 18, it would be a different matter—the ther-apist would have a duty to report this as child abuse. I then asked whether the total difference in the therapist's stance was whether the person harmed was under or over age 18. She replied, "Yes." For me, this is a substitute of law for ethics without understanding the moral underpinnings of the law itself.

This exchange reminded me of a clinical demonstration I heard by a famous therapist in the late 1970s. It was an interview of a married man dealing with an anxiety disorder and currently having an affair. The therapist worked his model of therapy with the man, including exploring the relation-ship between his anxiety and the affair. During the question-and-answer session after the recorded interview, an audience member noted that the wife and her stake did not come up in the session and asked why. The thera-pist responded crisply, "She's not my client." This reflects the individualistic bent of much psychotherapy: "My responsibility is only to the person in front of me in my office, with limited legal exceptions."

In fairness to the New York analyst and the famous therapist doing the demonstration, I can see that, absent a way to do sensitive, skilled ethical con-sultation (skills not taught in the field), entering the ethical domain with clients would threaten a core mission of therapy: to help clients make meaning of their actions and live self-determined lives. If the choice feels like being silent about (nonviolent) harm to others in clients' lives versus alienating and losing the client by judging and moralizing, it's probably better to remain silent and hope the client comes to make ethically sound choices through the normal process of therapy. But silence has its own costs. As mentioned in the Introduction, we are all meaning-making creatures who deal regularly with issues of right and wrong, of self-interest and responsibility to others. Psychotherapy is sapped of healing power if it ignores this ethical dimension of our clients' lives. There is no separating psychological well-being from the client's experience of having ethical integrity.

THE MANY CONTEXTS AND MEANINGS OF AFFAIRS

Some affairs are impulsive one-time encounters that the person regrets, doesn't disclose to the spouse, and decides never to repeat. These usually do not come up in therapy except perhaps as part of a personal sexual history. On the other end of the continuum are long-term affairs with someone who becomes a potential life partner. An even greater complication here is when this affair partner is close to the spouse. In between are brief affairs (sometimes multiple ones with different individuals) and ongoing affairs with someone who is not a potential mate. Then there are in-town variations that involve continual lying about one's whereabouts versus out-of-town affairs that involve more episodic deception.

Just as there are multiple kinds of affairs having different impacts on marriages, there are a variety of meanings that affairs have to those engaging in them. (Esther Perel, 2017, has done a particularly good job of articulating these meanings.) Meaning making in ethical consultation involves exploring the often-competing needs of self and others. "What does an affair do for me, and what are its consequences for my spouse and others?" Leaving off the first part would make the consultation shallow and ineffective. Notice in the Cheryl case how much I explored the meaning of her affair in terms of her experience of a dull marriage and a new sense of aliveness through the affair. Here are some different meanings an affair might have, framed in language a client might use:

- **That wasn't me.** "I was having a great time at a convention, got into drinking and dancing with someone attractive, and ended up in bed with her. This is not me. I feel awful about it and never told my wife."

- **Do I still have it?** "I was wondering whether I was still attractive and could feel sexually free like I used to feel. When that guy from work made a pass and asked me out, I said yes and had a great time."

- **I'm frustrated in this marriage.** "I don't feel connected or sexually fulfilled, so I go elsewhere."

- **I'm entitled to this.** "I have needs that can't be met in this or any marriage."

- **I need solace.** "My life is falling apart, and I need someone who can comfort me."

- **I am taking revenge.** "I'll get back at my partner who cheated on me."

- **The marriage is basically over.** "I'm done with this marriage even though we're still together, so why not see someone else?"

- **I need a way out of this marriage.** "I've wanted to leave for a long time. Maybe this relationship will give me the courage," or "I hope my spouse will end the marriage when this affair comes out."

Then there are the reactions of the spouse to the affair once it's revealed. These can include trauma, betrayal, fear, rage, and self-doubt, as well as milder responses when someone has been ready to end the marriage (Shackelford et al., 2000). Almost universally, there is a sense of hurt and anger about being deceived and lied to repeatedly. Some spouses say that the deception was worse than the sexual part. These reactions, real or potential when the affair is not yet known about, are important to fold into the client's meaning making about the affair and into the ethical consideration of the effects on the spouse.

STRATEGIES FOR ETHICAL CONSULTATION ABOUT AFFAIRS

I focus this discussion on ethical dimensions of working with married clients (or in a similarly committed relationship) who are currently having a secret affair. As with other case material described in this book, there are other clinical dimensions I do not discuss in any detail to concentrate on the less familiar ethical aspects. (Keep in mind that no therapeutic work involves only the ethical domain that I am focusing on here.) I outline the approach in terms of the LEAP-C (listen, explore, affirm, offer perspective, challenge) skills.

Listen

The key here is to listen for whether the client expresses guilt or remorse for the affair in terms of their value system and the effects of the affair on the spouse and others. For the most part, I've found that clients spontaneously express moral concerns about their affair—for example, "I never thought I would cheat on my wife," "I always saw myself as being faithful," "I feel great when I'm with her and then guilty when I come home," "I know this is unfair to my husband who thinks I'm a loyal wife." It's also important to hear when the client expresses no spontaneous remorse but instead stays with complaints about the marriage and what it has been like to live without sex, affection, and so forth. Because guilt is often intertwined with resentment toward the person we feel guilty about, sometimes all that comes out at first is the resentment ("Having no sex drove me to do this"), with guilt coming out later in the conversation.

Explore

When the client spontaneously expresses guilt or remorse about the affair, you can explore the meaning and other emotions involved. Unless the client is collapsing into self-loathing ("I'm a horrible human being and don't deserve to be married"), be willing to stay with the guilt as opposed to just noting it, normalizing it, and then immediately moving on to more comfortable therapeutic terrain: "When you say you feel bad about what you are doing to your marriage, could you say more? What effects do you see or worry about?"

The client may also worry about consequences for the affair partner, and this is also grist for ethical consultation. Perhaps the affair partner is also married or expects that the affair will lead to a long-term relationship that the client does not see happening. The moral foundations theory concepts of fairness and reciprocity come into play when the affair partner is kept in asymmetrical limbo. However, I recommend being careful about equating effects of the affair to those of a spouse who is usually in the dark about what's going on and has probably built a life around an expectation of sexual fidelity.

When the client's ethical concerns are fully part of the conversation, you can go back and forth between the meaning making about the affair (see the partial list earlier) and the ethical consequences. For example, you can explore the client's feelings of loneliness and sexual deprivation as a source of the affair and then switch to how the client feels about the solution to that problem via an affair that ends with remorse and other potential damage. Both sides of this are real: the meaning of the affair in the client's life (like divorce, affairs are often an attempted solution to a problem) and the consequences to self and others.

An important point is that I never suggest that the factors that led to the affair are a full justification for the affair. I frame them as influences and risk factors (such as a midlife crisis related to job loss and plummeting self-esteem) but not as determinants. The same with a sexless marriage, which is certainly a predisposing factor, but there are other ways to deal with the problem than launching an affair—for example, by starting couples therapy or even bringing up the idea of divorce if nothing changes. It's important that the therapist not accept that the client has no agency about the affair. It is a choice among other possible choices, given the circumstances of the client's life. No one "falls" into an affair, and no spouse "makes" their partner have an affair.

If a client has not expressed regrets or concerns about the consequences of the affair for the partner, you can ask questions to elicit that concern. I sometimes start with an empathic connection and then ask an ethical question: "I hear you on how unloved and frustrated you've been in your marriage, and that led you to have an affair. I also want to ask you whether having an affair is consistent with your values and how you see yourself."

Affirm

In my clinical practice, clients generally have said that cheating on their spouse compromises their values, that it's not who they are or want to be in their core. In some cases, this sense moves them to consider ending the affair, while in other cases, it moves them toward divorce (or ending a committed relationship) because they no longer want to feel morally compromised ("I don't want to live a double life anymore"). In either case, I affirm the client's sense of disjuncture between how they are living and how they believe they ought to be living: "I appreciate that you never thought you were the kind of person to go outside your marriage," or "I'm glad that you are thinking about how your wife is going to be affected when she finds out about your affair."

What if a client blames the spouse so much that they express no remorse or even ambivalence for their affair? In that case, I would ask about how they would feel if the partner spouse cheated on them and see whether that could generate a deeper conversation. My goal would be to open up the ethical domain of consequences of the client's actions for others and see whether I can affirm some semblance of ethical concern. If nothing else, I might be able to affirm that the client was here in therapy troubled enough to tell me about their affair. Openness with me is a start.

Perspective

Clients having affairs often need ethical perspective from their therapist, partly because affairs can be so emotionally powerful that balanced personal perspective is hard to come by. To emphasize again: The rhythm of the ethical consultation is to go back and forth between the client's emotions and meaning making about the affair, including what the affair is doing for them in a positive way (think of the Cheryl case) and the consideration of the effects on others. For the latter, here are perspective comments I often make when the client appears not to be seeing what is involved for their spouse. The craft here is to introduce these perspectives in a low-key rather than emphatic way.

- "You know, you're struggling with what to do while your husband is living with the illusion that there is no one else involved in his marriage."

- "I've learned that for a lot of people, the hardest part is realizing that they have been lied to over and over. They don't know what is real any longer. I imagine you can understand what that would be like."

- "In my experience, at some point, ongoing affairs tend to come out. When that happens, your wife will be in a world of hurt that you'll have to deal with in some way. I'm sure you have thought about this. I'm just putting it on the table."

Another technique is to invite the client to give themselves advice via an imagined third party. This often brings some clarity.

- "If you had a close friend in the same situation who asked you for input on what to do, what would you say?"

Then there are perspective statements related to the client's image of self as a moral person, an image that the affair often calls into question. Here are examples:

- "It's almost like there are two parts of you at war with each other now. One part is the ethical, loyal part that would not hurt anyone by having an affair, and the other part is saying, 'This relationship feels so good and is doing so much for me right now.' It can be hard to put those two parts together and figure out a direction."

- "I do think at some point you're going to have to make a choice about keeping your marriage or staying in your affair. There is a saying about a man with a foot in two canoes. They can stay together for a while, but at some point, they split apart and he's got to jump into one. I know this is hard."

A final perspective example is related to people's ultimate responsibility for their ethical choices. When a client continues to put most of the onus for the affair on the spouse's poor marital behavior, I say something like this:

- "I'd like to tell you how I see the ultimate responsibility for affairs. Even though there can be lots of factors that can lead to an affair—and we've discussed some of them in your marriage—at the end of the day, the decision to go outside the marriage belongs to the person who made that choice. The final responsibility is 100% on the person who had the affair, just as when someone physically hits their spouse, the responsibility for hitting is 100% on them even if the spouse said terrible things in an argument. If I choose to become violent instead of walking away or keep talking, that's on me. In the same way, nothing makes someone cheat on their spouse. That's my view on this. [*Pause*] Let me know your response."

I have found that this clarity on my end helps clients understand their agency and responsibility in a confusing situation: Both spouses share some responsibility for the chronic problems in a marriage, but the spouse who chooses the path of an affair is individually responsible for that action. The analogy to physical violence (again, delivered in a compassionate way) helps bring the message home: "My spouse may have provoked my anger, but I alone choose to slap or punch."

A final area of perspective giving is about whether to tell the spouse about the affair. This is a complicated matter that therapists differ on, with some believing in full disclosure of any affair, past or present, while others encourage not sharing. This came up in my interview with Cheryl presented earlier in this chapter. I don't have a definitive viewpoint on this matter because of the complexities of each couple's situation, but it's important for the therapist doing ethical consultation to have something meaningful to share with clients who seek input. Here is my perspective on disclosure.

On the end of the continuum are affairs of the distant past. I see little usefulness in doing what one elderly client did when he thought he was on his deathbed: tell his wife about an affair with a friend of hers 40 years ago. She was devastated and had trouble forgiving him after he recovered. I helped him see that although he felt a need to "confess" his transgression, it would have been better to share his secret with someone other than his wife.

On the other end of the continuum is a current affair that has threatened the survival of the marriage because the marriage was on shaky grounds, or the affair partner could have become a new mate. Knowing that the final decision is the client's, not mine, I am apt to support disclosure here so that the spouse understands a key reason the marriage was on the brink and can make an informed choice about whether to work on saving the marriage. Healing will be needed, hopefully in couples therapy, but at least there will no more secrets under the table.

Between those relatively clear cases, there is the murkier territory of disclosure that comes down to risks and benefits of full airing for those involved. The decision is up to the client. We offer perspective but do not get a vote.

Challenge

Sometimes, after spending a good deal of time using the LEAP skills (and after a good therapeutic alliance is in place), I decide to move from perspective to challenge on the issue of affairs. Recall the criteria for using ethical challenges: when the client has a big blind spot, is not seeing the immediate harm to someone, or is acting in a way inconsistent with their values. I recall a woman (Susan) who was having a torrid affair with a man who she described as sexy but "a dirtbag" in terms of personality, someone who said he adored her. She told me that her husband, who tended to be jealous, was getting suspicious. She knew what she was doing was wrong but didn't think she could reveal the affair and then keep a promise to end it. At a meaning-making level, it seemed clear that now middle aged and confused about the next stage of her life, she craved affirmation of being lovable and sexy. There was also an element of getting back at her jealous husband by actually cheating on him. I saw a train wreck coming for herself, her marriage, and her two children, who were benefiting from a stable family.

When delivering a challenge, I often begin by framing it in terms of worry for the client. In this case, "Susan, I'm worried for you right now. You've said that this affair is doomed because you don't really respect the guy, and there is a crisis coming if and when your husband finds out on his own. It feels like you are playing with fire here."

A similar challenge technique is to invite the client to imagine a future self who is looking back at the current self and the situation: "What would your future self say was the right thing to do?" (notice the use of the explicit ethical term "the right thing"). Even stronger would be "What do you want to be able to say to your children, if you and your wife divorce, about how you handled this critical moment in the life of their family?" I have found this last question particularly powerful when someone knows that they are not calling on their mature self at the moment, as in the case of a woman who was testing her husband's jealousy and potentially blowing up the family over a relationship with a man she did not respect.

It's important to end a challenge with a reaffirmation of the client's autonomy in making their own decisions. I sometimes say it this way: "I appreciate how you have taken a hard look at what's going on for you right now and that you've let me push you a bit. However you decide to move forward, I'll be here for you."

The final example relates to past affairs when the client does not accept responsibility for their choices, claiming instead that their spouse or an unhappy marriage forced them into the affair. They may say that they had pleaded with their sex-withdrawing or nasty spouse to change or go to therapy with them to no avail. The affair came inevitably out of that desperation. My challenge response: "I hear you that you tried and nothing changed. I also want to say that you could have ended your marriage at the point when you believed nothing would change. There are always other choices than having an affair that you acknowledge has compromised your values."

Infidelity is a quintessential ethical issue because it seriously affects the welfare of someone else. An ethically informed psychotherapy accepts the reality that once you've committed to being faithful to another person, your sex life and romantic life are not just your own. Working only with a perspective on the self-interest of the individual client limits the potential of psychotherapy to be a venue of healing and growth and in a larger way contributes to the erosion of communal bonds in society. Once we accept the notion of the relational self that inherently involves responsibilities to others, the challenge becomes how to incorporate this perspective into everyday practice in a caring, skillful, and seamless way that the clients experience as regular, helpful therapy and not some jarring switch into the territory of judgment and prescription. If this kind of integrated ethical consultation can be done with clients having affairs, it can be done with any client and any issue.

5
LYING AND DECEIVING

It was a brief moment in an ordinary therapy session with Lynn, a woman in her late 40s, who came to therapy to put her life back together after a difficult divorce.[1] She and her ex-husband had an exceptionally contentious coparenting partnership, marked by continual conflict and expensive lawyers. Lynn had gone through periods of refusing to have contact with Ron, her ex, making the children serve as the go-betweens. (This had been the topic of ethical consultation in our therapy, and Lynn was now communicating directly instead of putting the children in the middle.) She was now working on collaborating with Ron while maintaining her boundaries.

On this day, Lynn recounted with pride how she had handled her latest challenge with Ron. He texted her to say that his parents were coming to town on a weekend when Lynn was scheduled to have the children. They would love to spend time with the grandkids, he wrote, and the grandkids had not seen them for some time. Would Lynn be willing to trade weekends? Although Lynn told me that this particular request was reasonable, many

---

[1]The case examples in this chapter have been modified to disguise the identities of the clients involved and to protect their confidentiality.

https://doi.org/10.1037/0000263-006

The Ethical Lives of Clients: Transcending Self-Interest in Psychotherapy, by W. J. Doherty

prior ones had been at Ron's whim, and he had rarely been accommodating to her requests for a revised schedule. She had always bent when he put his request in terms of the children's needs (e.g., wouldn't they enjoy a ski trip that he could only book on a certain weekend?). Lynn told me that she decided not to go along with Ron this time, which, she noted, was her right under the divorce settlement.

Then she told me how she went about declining: by making up the excuse that she had already booked nonrefundable airplane tickets for an out-of-town trip with the children for that weekend. Ron immediately backed off his request, and Lynn was proud of herself. She had stopped him in his tracks and avoided the kind of pushback, insistence, and criticism she had gotten from Ron in the past. As Lynn moved on to a new topic in our session, I began pondering how I wanted to respond to her story. I knew I wanted to deal with her lie but needed a few moments to figure out how. A complication was that she felt good about her action and was not asking for my input on it, other than perhaps hoping for my affirmation.

I invite you to join me in deciding how to handle this moment. Therapists since the time of Freud have been more focused on clients' self-deception than their deception of others. But there was little obvious self-deception here: Lynn knew what she wanted to achieve and chose to create a fictional story to accomplish her goal. If you see yourself as an empowerment-oriented therapist, particularly with women like Lynn, who had been manipulated and controlled by her ex-husband, then perhaps you would see her response as a healthy sign that she was setting clear boundaries. Or perhaps you would see her deception as a risky way to set a boundary because the husband would eventually realize that no trip was going to occur, leading to a confrontation worse than if she had just said "no" at the outset, with no excuses.

Nowhere (that I know of) in the therapy literature is there a method of addressing this kind of situation on ethical terms. As I've said repeatedly, that's not been our familiar territory as therapists, even though what Lynn presented was a clear example of something that every culture and religion would see as a lie, something generally viewed as ethically concerning. The philosopher Sissela Bok (1979), one of few philosophers to address the social implications of lying, maintained that being able to count on the other's truthfulness is a foundation of social relations among human beings. It's the basis of trust, without which relationships and social institutions collapse. According to Bok, truthfulness does not mean saying what is true; it means saying what one believes is true. Lynn could have been mistaken about the dates of the ski weekend and thus been truthful in declining Ron's request.

A lie, according to Bok, is "an intentionally deceptive message in the form of a statement" (p. 33). It's telling you something I believe is untrue to deceive you. It's an active process rather than hiding something from you. If Lynn had said, "I'm not sure yet what our plans are for that weekend, and I don't want to give it away," she would not have been lying.

Lying, according to Bok, is different from maintaining one's privacy. Truthfulness does not require the revelation of all of one's feelings, thoughts, and experiences. When Lynn was asked to trade weekends, she did not have to reveal her reasons for not doing so: She could just decline (although Ron would likely have probed and pushed, which is why she made up a story). How much to reveal to another person depends on the relationship and the person's claim on that revelation. If Lynn and Ron were still married and Ron wanted to free up a weekend for his parents to visit, Lynn would have a responsibility to be transparent about her reasons for not wanting them to visit.

You might argue that Lynn had no obligation to refrain from lying to Ron because they were no longer married, and he was manipulative and coercive. If the problem with lying is that it erodes trust, in this case, there was little trust to erode. Maybe Lynn doesn't care whether Ron trusts her. Here is where Bok's second ethical dimension of lying comes into play: Deliberately deceiving someone puts a burden on them that they did not choose. It manipulates them by distorting their sense of reality. It induces them to act in ways against their interests. Stated differently, lying exercises power over someone who does not have a choice in the matter. In terms of moral foundations theory, this is about fairness versus cheating.

As mentioned, Lynn was not expressing any ambivalence about lying to Ron. It was a rare victory for her. Ethical consultation is easier when the client expresses ambivalence or regret about their actions. Before I describe how I handled this moment, I want to outline traditional ways of responding to the situation that avoid the ethical domain: (a) affirm Lynn's self-empowerment ("You stood up for yourself here"), or (b) offer a caution about the lie backfiring on Lynn herself ("How are you going to handle it when the weekend approaches and it becomes clear you are not leaving town with the kids?"). The first way implies that being trustworthy is not important in her coparenting relationship with Ron (therapists sometimes side so fully with divorced clients that they do not see an ex as having ethical claims in the coparenting relationship). The second way limits the scope of the conversation to the client's self-interest as if there are no other stakeholders in the decision to lie.

As just mentioned, Lynn gave me no hesitation or mixed feelings to connect to. While I reflected on how to respond, Lynn moved on to another topic related to parenting. I waited for an opening and returned to what she had said to her ex: "I'd like to go back for a moment to your text exchange with Ron about his request to change the weekend scheduling. Is that okay?" She said that was fine. Here is a re-creation of our exchange, with some commentary reflecting on the use of four of the LEAP-C skills: listen, explore, affirm, and offer perspective.

ME: It sounds like you accomplished your goal of keeping your boundaries on the parenting time schedule, given how flexible you've been in the past and how inflexible Ron has been. [I began by identifying with the self-interest part of the ethical issue. In terms of the LEAP-C skills, I had listened and was now exploring the meaning of Lynn's response in terms of her immediate goals.]

LYNN: Yes, that felt good for a change.

ME: I am wondering how you feel about making up a story to get him to back away. [Further exploring, I shifted to the other side of the ethical issue by naming it with soft language ("making up a story") and asking for her feelings about it. Notice the use of a soft I-message: "I am wondering" as opposed to a direct question, such as "Why did you . . .?"]

LYNN: [*Looking a bit rueful*] Yeah, it worked for the moment, but I'm not sure it was a good idea.

ME: Why not?

LYNN: For one thing, he may ask the kids about it as the weekend approaches and find out that we're not going on a ski trip.

ME: That makes sense. And what would be the fallout when the kids let him know? [I'm probing for the effects on Lynn and the kids as opposed to Ron.]

LYNN: Well, Ron will be furious, and I'll get a flurry of texts. And I'll be the bad guy again.

ME: Including with the kids?

LYNN: Yeah, they will be in the middle again and upset that they don't get either a ski trip or time with their grandparents.

ME: Lots of potential fallout from a made-up excuse. [This is a perspective statement from me, agreeing with Lynn's assessment.]

LYNN: Yep.

ME: So, what do you think led you to lie to Ron? [Here, I explore some more and introduce the explicitly ethical term "lie."]

LYNN: I felt bad about saying "no" and the kids not seeing their grandparents, but he has been so unfair about trading weekends when I want to. [Note that she is using ethical language to describe Ron's actions.]

ME: You know, I think you are selling yourself short. I think you can handle just saying "no" to Ron on something like this or even, if you choose, telling him that you are not inclined to trade because of his past unwillingness to trade with you. I think you are at the point where you could handle his reaction when you are being straight up. [This was a combination of affirmation and offering perspective.]

LYNN: I suspect you're right. I've created a mess by lying to get out of a sticky moment.

ME: It's understandable, given how run over you've felt so often in the past. I'm saying that you are stronger than that now, and you don't need to create such complications. What's that line? "Oh, what a tangled web we weave when first we practice to deceive."

LYNN: That's what happened here. A lesson learned. I don't need to do this.

This exchange engaged Lynn clinically and ethically: She could keep her boundaries and integrity. For me, the clinical and the ethical dimensions of therapy are seamless.

LYING AND DECEPTION IN PSYCHOTHERAPY

As mentioned earlier, the psychotherapy literature has been more concerned with self-deception than with lying to deceive others. The interpersonal aspects of lying among adults have been more the concern of social psychologists (who usually do experimental research to determine how various motivational and environmental factors influence people to lie; DePaulo, 2018) and of personality psychologists (who examine individual differences in the tendency to lie; Giluk & Postlethwaite, 2015). Overall, much more literature has focused on the development of honesty in children and adolescents than on lying and deception among adults.

What are the most common situations in which adults lie? Hart et al. (2019) articulated the following categories in their assessment of situational motivators for lying: protecting others, enhancing one's image, saving face, avoiding punishment, being vindictive, obtaining privacy, being entertained, avoiding confrontation, attaining instrumental gain, and maintaining and facilitating relationships. DePaulo (2018) reduced these categories to self-serving lies and other-oriented (or other-protective) lies, with the former occurring much more often than the latter. In terms of understanding how often adults lie, most studies before that of Serota and Levine (2015) studied samples of undergraduates. With their nationally representative sample of 1,000 U.S. adults queried about lies told in the past 24 hours, Serota and Levine found an average of one to two lies per day, with a wide range: 60% of people told no lies at all in the past day, and almost half of all lies were told by just 5% of individuals whom the authors referred to as "prolific liars." So, lying is common, the reasons are many, and some people lie a lot more than others.

In the world of mental health, chronic lying and deceit are considered pathological and potential markers of antisocial personality disorder. There is a literature on treating individuals whose lying reflects this kind of deep psychopathology (e.g., Gibbon et al., 2010). My interest here is how therapists address the ethics of lying among clients who understand the importance of honesty (they have a conscience) but who sometimes resort to lying as a way to avoid conflict, disapproval, embarrassment, or other reasons not connected to psychopathology.

From a humanistic psychology perspective, lying to maintain one's self-image or avoid interpersonal unpleasantness is a form of inauthenticity (Rogers, 1961). On this point, the philosopher Charles Taylor (1992) maintained that there is no contradiction between the authentic self and the honest self. Although there is a dark side to an emphasis on self-fulfillment, Taylor argued that there can be a moral ideal connected to self-fulfillment as being true to oneself. "Authenticity," he wrote, "points us towards a more self-responsible form of life" (p. 13). The argument here is that because we are inherently social creatures, being true to oneself means acting responsibly toward other people in one's life, which involves being truthful and not deceiving them. Being truthful creates trustworthiness in relationships, whereas deceiving others compromises relationships and eventually leads to inauthentic living based on not facing truths about oneself. Because the self is intrinsically relational, there is no sharp dividing line between intrapsychic truth telling and interpersonal truth telling.

Not that this kind of harmony between self and other is always easy to achieve in everyday life or therapy, as indicated by the following case of Nathan, where I got myself tied up in a secret that led to a failed therapy.

(Major secrets are usually maintained by lies.) Nathan was in his early 50s and divorced and came to me for help with problems with not maintaining an erection with his female partner. (He had never had this problem before.) I urged him to invite his partner to the first session, but he wanted to meet with me alone a couple of times to "get my head on straight." After a couple of sessions, his partner did come in, and before long, their sexual relationship was restored after Nathan learned to be more vulnerable and less performance oriented with a woman he genuinely loved, compared with the one-night-stand encounters he had experienced since his divorce.

A year after their wedding, Nathan called again, saying there were some things he had to sort out about himself and the relationship, and he wanted to begin with an individual appointment. He told me that he had been diagnosed with a heart–lung problem that would certainly limit his life expectancy. Even now, it was limiting his usual boundless energy. He was also having marital problems, feeling controlled by his wife's expectations of him. He had not told his wife about his diagnosis and prognosis and instead suggested that his decline in energy was related to his age and work demands. He wanted me to see him and his wife for couples therapy, and for now, he wanted to keep his medical condition confidential.

For me, the ethical part of this is that his partner had a stake in knowing what the future likely held for both of them, and she deserved to understand the true source of his lower energy now. When I raised a concern about his not telling his wife about his medical problem, especially if he wanted to work on improving the relationship, Nathan became agitated. She could not handle the news, he said. She would become too upset and worried about the future. (He was the family breadwinner.) If I had to do this case over again, I would have slowed down and taken a session or more to explore Nathan's fears of telling his wife and his feeling about lying to her about his condition. But instead of slowing down and exploring his dilemmas, I moved right into challenging him. I suggested that he might be responding to his fears about the future by trying to protect his wife. Knowing her as I did, I said I thought she could handle the truth and would prefer the truth. I said that she was in the same lifeboat with him and deserved to know that there were rapids ahead. Nathan pushed back hard, pleading and even insisting that I not make his telling her a condition for marital therapy. He offered a bargain with me: He would tell her after he figured out how to do so. Meanwhile, the relationship was in trouble, and would I please start the therapy? I relented, a decision I came to regret.

Why did I not slow down and explore what was going on for Nathan? I think I felt under pressure to decide whether to start the couples therapy as he was requesting. Therefore, I wanted the secret out now so that the couples therapy would be based on reality. This led me to skip over the early ethical consultation skills of exploration and offering perspective. Not surprisingly, I got a big push back and an urgent request to begin the work I know how to do—couples therapy. We started couples therapy, Nathan never told his wife, I held a secret in the couples therapy, and the therapy failed.

WHEN LITTLE LIES BECOME BIG LIES

So far, we've discussed big lies and deceptions where the welfare or needs of third parties are involved. This is in keeping with our working definition of the ethical realm in therapy: client behavior that has consequences for the welfare of others. But what about smaller lies, sometimes called "white lies," which are usually intended to avoid social embarrassment. One classic example is a response to your aunt's question about whether you like her hard-as-a-rock fruitcake. Most of us would respond, "Yes, Aunt Martha, it's delicious," instead of the more truthful "I don't care for it." The latter would be honest but cruel, and the harm of the little lie is minimal. A certain amount of withholding the truth is necessary as a lubricant for social inter-action, as when your colleague asks, "Could everybody see how nervous I was during my presentation?" "Yes, I'm sure they saw it," would not be a kind initial response. Bok (1979) warned that there is a slippery slope with white lies. If used too often, they can undermine one's reputation for veracity. And there is a difference between lying to protect someone else from social embarrassment and lying to protect oneself.

This difference between other-protective versus self-protective white lies came up with a couple in therapy. Marti and Emily, a lesbian couple, had been together for 2 decades and had two teenage children. In our session, they discussed their coparenting differences, one of which was about encouraging or discouraging white lies by their children. The latest example was the fol-lowing: Their oldest son Jeff, age 17, was scheduled to get an award at his high school. He mistakenly thought the dress code was casual. When he and his parents showed up for the event, at which he was to give a short speech, they realized that everyone else was dressed up, while Jeff was wearing jeans and a sweatshirt. Marti, his more open-to-white-lies mother, huddled with him about how to handle the situation. They came up with this strategy: Jeff would apologize to the audience for his attire, explaining that he had been serving food at a local homeless shelter and lost track of time before having to come directly to the school for the ceremony. The audience was impressed. Jeff had saved face, as had his family.

When Emily brought up this incident in a couples session, I asked them to discuss it as coparents. In their discussion, Marti carried the day by pointing out that Jeff's clothing misadventure was a minor mistake on his part and that no one was harmed by the story he told. In fact, he saved the audience from being embarrassed for him. No harm, no foul, Emily conceded, although she didn't like the pattern of white lies their kids were engaging in. On her end, Marti was proud that Jeff had come up with the creative story mostly on his own, with some enhancements from Marti.

After this period of helping them explore the context of what their son did, I affirmed them for respectfully airing their different feelings and views about the incident, without the kind of polarization that might have occurred in the past. After these affirmations, I went on to share two perspectives. I wondered whether Jeff might resort to making up excuses instead of facing the consequences of his mistakes in the future. I said that kids need real-world encounters with their mistakes, along with protection from harmful consequences. In this case, Jeff would have probably learned to pay more attention to dress expectations in the future.

Marti and Emily ended up not agreeing with my perspective about the award event scenario, and I did not move into the skill of challenging them because there was no immediate risk here. I did sense that Emily, in particular, took in what I had said. I ended by expressing one more concern about whether they would be able to believe their children as adults if they offered excuses for declining something such as an invitation for dinner. Would having to work late or having a minor ailment be believable or a way to say that they would rather not come to dinner on that particular day? They replied that they knew they could trust their kids. I had gone as far as I could.

Then, years later, this family came back in a crisis. Jeff was now engaged to marry a woman in a family that Marti and Emily knew well. All seemed fine until the younger sister (age 17) of Jeff's fiancée disclosed that Jeff had "made out" with her when they were alone a few weeks after the engagement was announced. When Jeff's parents confronted him about this, he denied it completely, saying that he had been visiting with his fiancée's sister (who he described as a dear young friend) and had an emotional conversation in which the sister had professed her love for him, but there had been no physical contact. Emily and Marti asked for an emergency family session with themselves and Jeff, who continued to deny there had been physical contact. I had doubts about Jeff's story, but he presented himself as appropriately sorry about his emotionally inappropriate relationship with his fiancée's teenage sister and putting himself into a compromising situation that created such stress for both families.

After I facilitated the family conversation in which there were tears and anger, Marti and Emily decided to believe Jeff's story, and the three of them went into damage control with Jeff's fiancée and her parents. The first goal was to preserve the wedding date 4 months out, which meant convincing the bride and her parents that although Jeff had made a mistake, there was no sexual abuse. There was also worry about the other family reporting Jeff to the authorities, even though at age 17, the sister was of legal age to engage in a sexual relationship with an older man.

After that emergency session, my involvement with the family ended for a time. Two months later, they came back after Jeff had confessed that the sister's story was correct. They had made out on the sofa in his fiancée's house. I explored with Jeff his story of a lifelong pattern of getting into tight spots and finding his way out of them with lies. I affirmed his willingness to take a deeper look at himself and referred him for individual therapy. There was no need for me to tell the parents, "I told you so." They saw it. The wedding was called off.

CHALLENGING LIES THAT COMPROMISE ANOTHER PERSON

As therapists, we are ethical consultants, not ethical gladiators. People are authors of their own lies. They can take our input or leave it, stay in therapy or drop out. But what do we do when a client seems to be lying boldly in a way that is destructive for someone in their life?

I was seeing Malcolm and Dottie for a shaky marital relationship. Malcolm admitted to prior affairs and claimed he was faithful now. Dottie was suspicious that he was seeing another woman. It was hard to get the therapy off the ground with this level of suspicion and pleading of innocence. I told them that I am not a detective or a judge and that I don't do couples therapy when there is an active affair. The alternatives were to either accept the premise that Malcolm was not seeing another woman so that we could work on their other problems, or Dottie could hold onto her sense of what was happening, and we would suspend couples therapy for now. (I tried to do this in a way that did not disconfirm Dottie's fears.)

Dottie decided that it was worth accepting Malcolm's word for now and embark on working on long-standing conflicts in the marriage. Malcolm was relieved and said he was ready to work on the relationship. However, it was slow going, with Malcolm, in particular, not signing up for any of his contributions to the problems. Dottie then brought up more worries about infidelity because he was gone from home so much without believable reasons. We were back in the morass of accusations and defense, a therapy spot I was not willing to stay in for long. Then came a session that Dottie attended alone; Malcolm said he had to cancel at the last minute because of a work commitment. Dottie brought a recording on her iPhone of a romantic-sounding conversation between Malcolm and another woman, with music in the background, which she received one afternoon in what appeared to be a mistaken "pocket call" from her husband.

At our next session, Dottie confronted Malcolm with this recording. He looked stunned and grew silent. I invited Dottie to leave the room and asked him about what she said and recorded. He looked at me straight and said calmly that she was wrong: He had been to an afternoon movie and had inadvertently placed that call during a romantic scene in the movie. He had not been with another woman

I didn't believe him. After using the LEAP skills in prior sessions, now I decided to use challenge without coming across as a scold or someone with authority over him—like a boss or a police officer who could wield consequences. I collected myself and told him how I felt:

ME: Malcolm, I'm having trouble believing you right now.

MALCOLM: Bill, I'm telling you it's all a big mistake. I was at a movie.

ME: I hear you. It's just that I can't find a way to accept what you're saying as the truth.

MALCOLM: But it is the truth.

ME: Again, I get what you're saying. It's just that I am having a hard time accepting it. I do know that I can't go forward with you in this therapy unless we have an agreement on what is true about you seeing another woman. It sounds like we don't have that agreement.

MALCOLM: I guess that means the therapy is over.

ME: Yes, I think it does. If you ever want to talk about all of this in the future as an individual, I'm available.

MALCOLM: Okay, I appreciate that.

ME: I'd like to bring your wife back in now and summarize our conversation, if that's okay with you, and to say why we're ending the couples therapy. Then I'd like to talk with her alone to finish up.

MALCOLM: Okay.

I learned to have this kind of challenging yet respectful conversation from coaching primary care clinicians to deal with patients who the clinician believes are lying about the medication or drug misuse—sometimes despite definitive laboratory findings to the contrary. The key is to "stay in your own lane" with what you can believe or not believe or what you have observed or not observed. Do not try to talk the client into changing their story, and do not attack the client's character or motives. It's best to do this with a tinge of regret that you and the client don't see this the same way; this helps you not come across as accusatory. Generally, clients in these situations have years of experience with lying, at least about certain aspects of their lives, such as using drugs or infidelity, and are used to clinicians being either gullible or authoritarian. They have standard responses for either but not for a firm, respectful, and boundaried response from the clinician.

Lying is most often motivated by self-protection and fear of retaliation—fully human and understandable impulses—but it comes with power over others. Being truthful when we feel pulled to lie is about vulnerability and sharing power. Although all the traditional models of psychotherapy support the value of truthfulness for the well-being of individual clients, for the most part, they overlook the importance of truthfulness in the moral order of relations between people. If therapists fail to see the ethical dimension of being truthful, we may end up only helping people speak the truth when it will serve their immediate needs or promote their personal growth. In a consumer world of transactional relationships, lying can easily become a strategically wise choice, as we see played out in the political realm every day. But the reality for us as social beings is we cannot be true to ourselves if we are not true with others.

6 HARMING OTHERS

When I've solicited written case examples of challenges therapists face in dealing with ethical issues in the lives of clients, at the top of the list of worrisome cases are those involving direct and immediate harm to others or the direct risk of doing harm. The damage can be physical or emotional, or both. Often, therapists worry about how their clients are harming children, but sometimes, as in the following case I was consulted about, it's other adults being put at risk without their knowledge and consent. To be clear: I am addressing harm in a broader way than how the therapy literature has traditionally engaged the question of harm as legal responsibility to report abuse or the duty to warn someone when a client makes violent threats about that person.

The therapist was seeing Brantley, a 30-something man who had been on the streets and in and out of drug rehabilitation programs for years.[1] Life had been hard for him, beginning with an abusive mother who eventually gave him up to the foster care system. A big guy with street smarts and charm, he had found ways to stay alive and keep a variety of women in his

---

[1]The case examples in this chapter have been modified to disguise the identities of the clients involved and to protect their confidentiality.

https://doi.org/10.1037/0000263-007
The Ethical Lives of Clients: Transcending Self-Interest in Psychotherapy, by W. J. Doherty

life as sexual partners, if not lovers. Now Brantley found himself infected with HIV, which he believed he had contracted from a woman. All of his rage against women, stemming initially from his relationship with his mother, now came to the fore, along with bouts of serious depression that led his physician to refer him for therapy.

The first therapy session was a safe place for Brantley to ventilate his anger toward women. His therapist later told me that he found Brantley's rage against women disconcerting but not too far out of the ordinary for a therapist used to working with volatile, needy men like Brantley. Then, Brantley announced his intention to have sex with as many women as possible to give them AIDS. He didn't just say he felt like doing this—he was intent on doing this, starting today. The therapist knew that Brantley had several current sexual partners and could readily find more. It should be noted that this was the time before effective treatment for this disease—it was a likely death sentence.

The therapist was alarmed and paralyzed about what to say or do next. He could not fall back on the therapist's duty to warn because none of the women were identified. He could see just two choices: (a) try to engage Brantley in a therapeutic exploration of his rage against women and hope he decided not to put women in his life at mortal risk or (b) tell him that what he is planning is wrong and he should reconsider. The downsides of the long-term approach were that Brantley planned to begin his antiwoman campaign immediately, and there was no way to know whether he would return for more therapy sessions. The risk of the second approach was that Brantley would react negatively to the admonition and drop out of therapy, leaving the therapist with no leverage because the duty to warn mandate was not applicable, given that the threat was general, not about any specific individuals.

The therapist took the first path: explore, empathize, build a relationship, and hope the client would pause and reconsider harming others. Unfortunately, Brantley did not return for another session, and the therapist never knew what became of the plan to infect as many women as possible. In case consultation, the troubled therapist's peers told him he had done all he could do. To confront his client in the first session, they maintained, without building rapport and delving into the roots of his hatred was not what therapists should do. Admonishing the client about his bad motives is what a pastor or a parent might do, but not a therapist.

Cases like Brantley's forever haunt therapists. Having come to a workshop on ethical consultation with clients, his therapist wanted to know whether there were alternatives he could have employed, knowing that he had done all he knew how to do at the time. I told him that I had never been in that situation and don't know how I would have responded. But reflecting now, without the urgency and pressure of the moment, I offered the following thoughts on how I might handle this situation using the LEAP-C skills (listen, explore, affirm, offer perspective, challenge) of ethical consultation.

I would begin with empathic listening about the anguish Brantley was feeling with his AIDS diagnosis and fear of illness and death. I would explore the pain that Brantley had experienced at the hands of women in his life. I would ask whether a woman (maybe a sister, a good foster mother, or his young daughter whom he did not see often) had been good to him amidst the hurt he experienced from others. I would explore whether he had perhaps done something good for a woman in his life—someone he protected from harm from another man, perhaps. In this last part, I would be searching for even one incident of moral good done for him or by him with regard to a woman—something I could delicately underline and affirm. (I doubted that he could have had so many women in this life as sexual partners if he were not capable of some kindness and care.) If Brantley were receptive thus far, I would then offer a perspective on his current plan to infect women. I might say that while I could understand why he would want to punish the women who had hurt him, I was puzzled by why he would want to harm so severely a number of women who had not hurt him.

All of these tactics, of course, are standard therapy approaches that I imagine Brantley's therapist tried. (The exception might be how I searched for a way to affirm his positive moral behavior toward some women.) In consulting with Brantley's therapist, I wanted to make sure I indicated the common practices I would have used first with Brantley, lest where I would go next seemed not based on a foundation of connection, exploration, and perspective. It's important not to jump immediately to where I would go next, even when the risk of harm is urgent.

If Brantley did not soften on his threats, I would challenge him, going back and forth between empathic and challenging statements. Because this was not my case, I won't use the client's part of the dialogue, just my part—knowing what I would say would depend on his responses. Here, then, are some sample lines I might use:

- "Brantley, I think I'm starting to understand how you are feeling about having HIV and why you are thinking about infecting and probably killing as many women as you can. This is a big moment for you, and I'm glad you have told me what you're planning. [Wait for his nonverbal response.] Can I push back at you on something right now?" [This last question is a skill I call *pivoting*, asking permission to offer a challenge before proceeding.

If the client agrees, as they almost always do, they are more prepared for what you say next. It also communicates respect for the client's boundaries. In this case, with a man who sees himself as tough, I would deliberately use the term "push back at you," which would almost certainly yield a "yes" response—he would see himself as able to handle my challenge.]

- "I'm really worried for you now. I think you are about to cause a lot more pain for yourself by hurting innocent people." [A first-level challenge can be about harm to self through remorse from hurting others.]

- "You wouldn't be here telling me about doing this unless you had at least a little bit of doubt. Heck, you could be in bed with a woman right now, passing on the AIDS virus. But you're here with me telling me about your hurt and anger." [This attributes ambivalence and conscience to the client. After all, he came voluntarily and opened up about his plan.]

- "I'm going to ask you some hard questions right now. Feel free to tell me to back off or go to hell. [Forecasting the challenge to prepare the client, inviting his courage, and affirming his autonomy.] Who is the woman or girl you care about the most on this planet? [Elicit a name based on the prior part of the conversation.] Okay, think about her. Imagine there is a guy out there who knows her. He has been hurt by women just like you've been hurt and is now thinking of punishing the women in his life, maybe by raping and beating them. He opens up to you about his plan, not realizing that you know a woman he might hurt. What would you say to him?" [If the client were with me, I would invite him to elaborate on what he would say and why. I'm encouraging his moral empathy, beginning with one woman.]

- "Brantley, I'm pushing you pretty hard on this. How is this going down with you? You can tell how concerned I am for you and for the women you know." [Another pivot to get his buy-in for the next all-out challenge.]

- "You didn't deserve what so many women in your life have done to you, and now, I want to say that the women in your life now don't deserve what you are thinking of doing to them. That's how I see it." [Once you've made a direct ethical statement like this, don't defend it if the client challenges it. Just calmly affirm that it's how you see the situation. The client is free to accept, reject, or continue to mull your stance, but don't debate it. You are modeling self-differentiation here: having an ethical viewpoint without being distressed if the client does not buy it.]

An analogy I might use if he seemed open to it is:

> You know, since we've been sitting here, I've been having this image of you like Samson. Remember him from the Bible? The strongest man in the world, and you look pretty strong to me. Do you recall that he was screwed over by a woman named Delilah, who cut his hair when he was asleep? He had reason to be furious only at her, but eventually, he brought down a temple and killed himself and a lot of innocent people. I'd love for us to work on you recovering from the Delilahs in your life and deal medically and emotionally with your HIV and not have all that collateral damage to other people. Maybe I didn't get the Bible story right, and maybe you think this was a silly way to describe you and your situation, but it's been in my head while we've been talking, Mr. Samson. [I would be reading his nonverbals to see how much in sync we are. I'm hoping for laughter at this point.]
>
> [If he is still tracking] I appreciate how you've let me push you. Are you up for meeting again? [If yes] I wonder whether we can make a deal: that you don't act yet on having unprotected sex until we have another conversation. In the meantime, you and I both can think about what we've talked about today. What do you think?

There are no guarantees about the outcome of this kind of intervention. I present it to illustrate how a therapist can stay in the role of therapist while offering ethical challenges to a client—an approach that respects the client's autonomy while calling on the client's moral sensibilities about harming others.

DIVIDED LOYALTIES AND RISK OF HARM

Brantley's temptation was to harm people based on past hurts. Other times, the ethical dilemma related to harm stems from current dilemmas, such as loyalty to one's spouse versus one's child from a previous relationship. Indeed, stepfamily life is like a mini-morality play with competing loyalties. I think of a client who felt pulled to spend every evening helping her children with their homework while her new husband wanted couple time. This is a relationship challenge but also an ethical dilemma of how to manage competing interests and obligations.

This kind of stepfamily dilemma came in a dramatic fashion in one of my most memorable cases.[2] A husband and wife, Phil and Marla, and I were

---

[2]This case example is from "Divided Loyalties: The Challenge of Stepfamily Life," by W. J. Doherty, 1999, *Psychotherapy Networker*, (May/June), pp. 33–38 (https://dohertyrelationshipinstitute.com/wp-content/uploads/2019/11/stepfamilies.pdf). Copyright 1999 by The Psychotherapy Networker, Inc. Adapted with permission.

in the winding down phase of marital therapy that had focused on how the couple could maintain their emotional connection while coparenting the husband's two teenage children, Nathan (age 15) and Kristin (age 18), whose birth mother lived out of state and had infrequent contact with her children. Marla had no children of her own. Kristin's adolescence had been tumultuous, with regular temper flare-ups at her father, which increased dramatically when he got involved with Marla. Although Kristin had settled down somewhat in her senior year of high school, she was still unpredictable in her moods. What's more, as her behavior improved, her younger brother took her place as the family's lead source of conflict.

Although Phil and Marla had come to me for marital therapy, I invited the children to come for several sessions because coparenting was such an issue. I saw firsthand how intense and challenging the kids were. They were uninterested in working on improving a stepfamily situation they had not signed up for. Neither of them was willing, when I talked to them alone, to get into their feelings about their mother's abandonment and their attitudes toward their stepmother, whom they barely tolerated. Any changes in the family would have to come from Phil's and Marla's initiative, not from any direct efforts on the part of the children.

By the ending phase of the yearlong couples therapy, Kristin had gone away to college, and the father and stepmother had learned to mesh their coparenting roles better. Marla had moved into a supportive, less critical role regarding Phil's parenting, and he was taking a firmer stance with his children by insisting that they show respect for Marla. There had been slow, steady progress on the kids' behavior, although Marla still felt tense in the home. With their marriage on solid footing for the first time, we started to wind down our therapy work.

Then a marriage-breaking issue surfaced. In the difficult early months of the marriage, Phil had promised Marla that once his children left for college, they would be on their own. They would be expected to find their own place to live, with their father's financial support, while they were in school. In other words, after high school, they could stay as family visitors but not as members of the household. This agreement kept Marla's hope alive during the darkest days of stepfamily life with teens. But the agreement was never shared with Kristin and Nathan.

During her visit home at the Christmas break of her first year in college, Kristin told her father she wanted to come home for the summer and find a job. Phil replied that he wasn't sure and would give her a decision later. This precipitated a meltdown by Kristin, who accused her father of abandoning her. Until that point in the visit, Kristin's behavior had been better than when she was in high school, but her emotional adjustment to college had been shaky, and now she became surly and shaken.

Phil's hesitation also elicited a strong response from Marla. In our therapy session, Marla said that she could not spend another summer with Kristin. Marla believed she had done enough. She had given herself over to an impossible stepparent role, had put up with disrespect, and had learned to be a supportive coparent and temper her criticism of her husband's parenting. She felt her health had been compromised because her migraine headaches were worse than before she got married. She did not think she could face another summer of stress with Kristin. She wanted Phil to keep his promise. Although 15-year-old Nathan was a handful, at least he was just one child, and he would be gone in 3 years too. Marla felt betrayed when Phil hesitated to follow through on their deal.

For his part, Phil was torn. He knew he had made the promise to his wife and understood how much she had been awaiting this leaving-home stage, but he felt an obligation to take Kristin back when she wanted to come home. Phil did not want her to feel rejected by him, especially after her mother had walked out of her life. And he wanted another chance to be a better parent, based on what he had learned in therapy. He wanted to make the summer period a healthier one for his relationship with his daughter, including starting with clear expectations that she would line up a job before coming home and would be a better citizen of the family. As he spoke, Phil got to his deepest fears in this situation: that he would either harm his daughter or lose his wife.

For me, at the end of a difficult but seemingly successful course of therapy, this was a most unwelcome impasse. A marriage that 4 weeks ago had been at its peak was now in the pits. They were looking to me to help them break the impasse at a time when I was prepared to make my goodbyes. This kind of family-splitting dilemma had not come up in my training. It was not in the textbooks. I never saw it in a master video case. Then I thought, "This is a moral dilemma. I am supposed to know how to work with this kind of thing. This is my specialty." The self-talk did not help. At the end of the session where all of this material came out, I ended lamely with something like, "I feel your pain; why don't you keep talking about it?" I hoped that in 2 weeks, they would make some progress on their own because I was stumped.

By the next session, they were even more dug into their positions. If Kristin returned home, Marla would feel deeply betrayed, fearful for her health, and probably leave the marriage. If Kristin did not return home, Phil would feel as if he had betrayed his daughter. (Note here the moral foundations theory intuitions of loyalty/betrayal and care/harm.) Marla did not believe she was asking her husband to betray his daughter. Kristin would be better off, she argued, if she stayed in an apartment near her out-of-state college; returning home would be a regression for a young adult. Phil felt otherwise and could not bring himself to turn down his 19-year-old daughter's request to come home for the summer.

From my perspective, Marla and Phil loved each other and had learned to resolve most of their conflicts. Neither of them seemed to be using this impasse for leverage in the marriage. They were just stuck. At first, I saw myself as neutral about the decision on whether Kristin should be allowed home for the summer. I saw good arguments on both sides, and I helped each spouse clarify their positions and the feelings that underlay them. I asked about the effects of a yes or no decision on everyone involved: Kristin, Marla, Phil, and Nathan. As I listened, I reflected more on Kristin, especially her carryover emotional fragility from being abandoned by her birth mother. I heard more clearly Phil's belief that he wanted another chance to do better by her as her father. And as I listened harder to Marla, I took in her fear of never having a marriage and household without oppositional offspring present.

In the end, I was no longer neutral. I believed that Phil owed his daughter an open door in the summer, given her history and current vulnerability. I tilted the discussion toward finding a way for Kristin to come home for the summer and Marla not to feel betrayed. I began surfacing the ethical issue involved: "Phil, if I am hearing you right, this comes down to a moral issue for you: You cannot live with yourself as a parent if you turn Kristin away this summer." Phil teared up, saying, "Yes, it is, but I feel so terrible about hurting Marla."

When I used the word "moral," Marla nearly jumped out of her seat. She could sense the tide turning because her case was not based on something as lofty as conscience but more on her self-preservation. I was prepared instantly to address her side. I said,

> And for you, Marla, I don't think this is really about whether you can survive the summer emotionally and physically. You have survived the past 3 years, and you are a resilient person. In fact, Kristin's behavior toward you is better than it has been in the past. There is no doubt in my mind that you can handle the stress of a summer stay. What I sense is that the deeper issue is whether you can trust your husband to keep his word and whether you can have any hope for a time when there are not children in the household, a time when you can feel the home is yours and your husband's.

Now, Marla, having been heard, teared up.

They were both listening carefully now. I went on to take even more focus off the summer decision, saying to Phil,

> If I were Marla, I would wonder whether you will ever be able to say "no" to one of your children who wants to move home. When they are 35 and would like a place to crash for a year to save money, could you turn them down? Can Marla ever count on a time when it will be just the two of you?

Marla interjected, "Yes, that's the main point. It is not mainly about this summer. It's about what this summer means for the future, about whether I can count on you to set limits on your children's role in our marriage."

Notice in this interaction that after using terms that elicited and validated Phil's moral position on the decision and thereby clearly moving my weight to his side, I immediately sided with Marla on what I thought were her deep and legitimate concerns. I introduced moral ideas such as trust and loyalty from Marla's side, giving her credit for more than blatant self-interest (wanting to be rid of the kid). I focused the issue away from the summer agreement toward their overall marital contract for the presence of Phil's children in their lives.

My challenge about his long-term loyalties moved Phil to affirm that he would never tolerate a willy-nilly use of the home by his adult children and that he too looked forward to being just a couple. It was just that this summer, he felt he could not say no, given Kristin's shaky first year away and her experience with her birth mother. When Marla, with less conviction this time, repeated her view that it would be best for Kristin not to come home, I offered my perspective. I said that the first summer home after leaving for college was a developmentally unique time. Many young people need to know there is a home to return to before they try their wings. I told them that I have seen parents make the mistake of turning the children's bedroom into a den the day they leave for college. One divorced parent I knew did that, and her daughter never stayed a night in her mother's house again, preferring to stay in her old room at her father's house. Furthermore, from what I knew of Kristin and her first year at college, she was still working through her angry dependence on her father and would take a "no" as a powerful rejection.

Notice here that I was tilting again toward Phil's position, so I quickly moved to affirm Marla's perspective by challenging Phil:

> What I hear from you, Phil, is that you don't want Kristin to come home for business as usual but that you are going to use this summer to work on your relationship with your daughter, including her contributions to the morale of everyone in the household.

Phil repeated his wish to have one more try at being a different parent to Kristin and his determination to do it better.

With the impasse softening but no solution emerging, I made a cautious proposal for them to think about, something that carried risks for both of them. This summer, they would agree that Phil could decide whether Kristin could come home, but in the future, it would require two votes: Phil's and Marla's. Marla immediately liked the idea, saying that she would not use her "veto" unless she thought the children were using the household as a revolving door. Phil said he would not want a revolving door either and that he looked forward to being alone as a couple. But the proposal was scary to him, and he needed time to think about it.

When we met for our final session, Phil announced he had agreed with the proposal and that coming to place this kind of trust in Marla had led to a breakthrough in their relationship. Marla herself was beaming even though Kristin was going to come home for the summer because she felt the partnership was restored. I told them how relieved I was and how worried I had been for them and Kristin. In the moments of celebration at the end of the session, I also told them I was relieved that a year's worth of effort on my part did not go down the toilet! I scolded them in jest for making me work so hard at the end of therapy.

This family had nearly fractured over conflicting loyalties. Because I saw Kristin as the most vulnerable stakeholder, the one at the most risk of harm, I took responsibility to influence the decision so as not to compromise her well-being. I also supported Phil's moral sense that he could not betray his daughter's fundamental needs, even to save his marriage. And I supported Marla's stake in being able to have a say in the future composition of her household and hope realistically for a postparental phase of family life.

I don't usually propose a specific resolution of clients' ethical dilemmas, but in this case, I made a proposal because I thought they could use something specific to think about. I was not attached to this particular way to resolve the impasse. But I was attached to the idea of preserving the marriage if possible, protecting Kristin, and helping both Phil and Marla meet their needs and keep their integrity. No wonder I was so relieved at the end; the combination of those outcomes is not easy to achieve in any family, let alone a struggling stepfamily.

WHEN CLIENTS HARM ADULTS IN THEIR LIVES

I want to reemphasize what's hard for therapists when it comes to client behavior that affects other adults in their lives. When it comes to children's welfare, most therapists are on board, in principle if not in the use of the skills, with taking steps to prevent harm. Law backs this up when there is abuse. But when an adult is the one at risk of harm, I think therapists are more ambivalent or even reluctant to speak up, except in situations such as flagrant abuse or threats, such as in the case of Brantley. And there, the full range of LEAP-C skills is even more important to be challenging without losing the client. Years ago, a colleague told me about being fired by his client after switching from a therapy based mainly on emotional support to telling the client in a particular session that he should stop acting in a manner that likely felt threatening to his ex-girlfriend. A good thought experiment is how you feel about a client's behavior toward a reviled ex-spouse. Examples include finding manipulative ways to get more than one's agreed-on share of parenting time, foisting additional child expenses on the other parent, or spreading negative information to friends and family members about the ex's new lover. Let's imagine that none of these actions directly affects the children; the client, for example, is not talking with the children about the ex's new lover, and the children are not losing out on expenses or missing lots of time with the other parent. In this scenario, the one mainly being manipulated or put upon is the ex-spouse. Do we as therapists feel any responsibility to question unfair treatment of a hated ex-spouse? That's a litmus test for ethical consultation.

Here's an example. Lenny, a client in my men's therapy group, was having a hard time managing his three young children in his small apartment when he had them every other weekend. When one of his children could not make a weekend, Lenny discovered that it was much easier to have just two children rather than three. He came to the group announcing with pride his breakthrough idea that he would change the parenting arrangement so that he would only have two of his children at a time. When one of the group members asked why his wife would go along with that idea because she would then never have a free weekend, he said he was confident she would agree if he framed it as being in the best interests of the children. "She is a sucker for the best interests of the children," he told us. The group seemed supportive of his strategy, which he said he planned to bring up to his ex that night.

I invite you to ponder what you would say or not say at this moment. Do you have a responsibility as a therapist to speak up about Lenny's plan, and if so, on what grounds? If you decide to intervene, how would you do it? What words would you say? How would you open up the ethical consultation?

Given the group's support for Lenny's plan, his intention to pitch it right away, and the limited amount of time each member of the group gets for their therapeutic work, I decided to move directly into the issue by asking the quintessential ethical question: "How do you think never having time free from parenting would affect your ex-wife?" Lenny quietly replied that it would probably be hard on her.

At that point, a strong pushback came from another member of the group, who happened to be a physician. Sitting next to me, he leaned toward me with a look of puzzlement: "Wait a minute, Bill. I don't get this. Lenny is your patient, not his wife. Those of us in this room are your patients, not people out there." That was a singular moment in my career. It brought from me an explanation of how I see my role as a therapist:

> I hear your surprise. I do see my first responsibility being toward you in this room. However, I have to be concerned about the welfare of others in your life, including those who are affected by what you do. In this case, I am concerned that Lenny's ex-wife might be manipulated into making a decision that will negatively affect her because she will have no time off from being a single parent. And eventually that will affect the children too.

Lenny immediately accepted what I said, agreeing that what was bad for his ex would be bad for the kids too. I also had the sense that he knew he was in the same coparenting canoe with his ex and that he owed her more than manipulating her. The client who challenged me seemed to accept my rationale. The group then rallied to find ways to help Lenny cope better with his three children at the same time. Two experienced single fathers in the group offered him their perspectives and willingness to advise him in the future. It was the first time I directly articulated my philosophy of ethical consultation directly in a therapy session.

This discussion sets up the next chapters on the self of the therapist as ethical consultant. How do the ethics and character of the therapist affect how we avoid or address the ethical concerns that clients bring to us? What is our sphere of responsibility? Chapter 7 addresses this question in terms of the self of the therapist, and Chapter 8 addresses it in terms of the public dimensions of psychotherapy.

PART **III** THE RESPONSIBILITIES
OF THERAPISTS AS
ETHICAL CONSULTANTS

7 THE SELF OF THE THERAPIST IN ETHICAL CONSULTATION

As in all healing professions, the person of the therapist is at the vital center of the work. Much of the literature on the self of the therapist focuses on how to become aware of the distortions we bring from our past that can limit our effectiveness with clients—our biases, blind spots, and unresolved personal issues that interfere with our work (e.g., Timm & Blow, 1999). At first glance, traditional self-of-the-therapist principles seem to run counter to the central argument in this book, namely, that the therapist does and must bring a moral sense to the therapeutic relationship. Influenced by Carl Rogers (1990) and others, most therapists expect to hold unconditional positive regard for their clients, a stance that Rogers argued "is at the opposite pole from a selective evaluating attitude—'you are bad in these ways, good in those'" (p. 225).

There is less inconsistency, however, if we make a distinction between being judgmental toward clients and discerning how their actions are affecting the welfare of other people in their lives. Being judgmental implies a negative attitude toward the client as a person in a way a therapist might feel about a political leader who is seen as duplicitous. However, if that political leader were to become our client, we would have to work to understand any current

https://doi.org/10.1037/0000263-008
The Ethical Lives of Clients: Transcending Self-Interest in Psychotherapy, by W. J. Doherty

unethical behavior in light of the person's larger life narrative and remind ourselves that no one can be defined by the worst things they have done. However, relating in a nonjudgmental way toward this politician client as a person would not mean having no views on the effects of the client's actions. Nor, from my perspective in this book, would it mean refraining from trying to influence this client in the direction of more ethical treatment of others in the future.

In sum, the challenge for the therapist as an ethical consultant is to accept clients as persons, flaws and all, while being willing to try to influence their behavior in the ethical realm. The latter is a traditional taboo in the therapy field. In other chapters, I've dealt with this apparent dilemma from a conceptual point of view, arguing that when clients bring ethical dilemmas to us (e.g., divorce vs. work on the marriage), we inevitably influence the client's decision-making process. In an individualist culture in which psychotherapy is practiced in the Western world, we imagine that we are being value free and morally neutral when supporting a client to mainly emphasize self-interest in the face of this ethical dilemma ("If you're not happy in the marriage, why are you staying?"). Once we recognize our inevitable influence in the moral zone of clients' lives, the question becomes not whether but how we use our influence—ideally with sensitivity and skill.

This chapter explores how therapists can become effective ethical consultants via three avenues: ethical self-awareness, cultural self-awareness, and an ethic of caring for other people whose lives intersect with those of our clients. I also return to the theme of the relational, committed self (Chapter 1) as it plays out for therapists in our lives.

THERAPIST SELF-AWARENESS IN THE ETHICAL REALM

Understanding oneself is the heart of any self-of-the-therapist perspective. In the realm of ethical consultation, I see self-awareness coming in two main areas: recognizing our moral intuitions that arise during interactions with clients and recognizing the origins or roots of these intuitions. This is where moral foundations theory (Haidt & Joseph, 2007) can be particularly helpful because it deals with both spontaneous moral feelings and the cultural roots of these feelings.

To review, the five moral intuitions in moral foundations theory are (a) care/harm, (b) fairness/cheating, (c) loyalty/betrayal, (d) authority/subversion, and (e) purity/degradation (see Chapter 1 for more details). They are not considered abstract philosophical categories but immediately accessible, affect-laden intuitions that we may subsequently try to understand cognitively and explain. The ethical situations about which we have intuitions extend beyond our self-interest—for example, my response when I notice someone cheating on me is, "Hey, that's not fair!" If someone cuts into a long queue behind me (not ahead of me), I am likely to have an immediate negative reaction to their cheating, even though it does not affect me directly. If asked to explain my reaction, I would have to search for the right words, perhaps ranging from "That is not fair to the others who have been waiting" to something about how the social order depends on people following basic rules of reciprocity. But my instantaneous response ("Hey, that's cheating!") came without any prior self-explanation. Of course, there is a cultural context here; there are places where line jumping is normative—just not in Minnesota, where I live!

I invite you to pay attention to the moral intuitions that arise in you when you read about the following case.[1] In a stepfamily where the children are living with their widowed father and his new wife of several years, there has been a lot of yelling and conflict between the spouses, much of it related to coparenting the husband's three teenage children and the birth of a new child who has a developmental abnormality. You are seeing the couple, and they recount a painful scene: The couple sat down with the 15-year-old girl to tell her that she has to start being more cooperative. She retorts that they are not being fair to her. The stepmother then begins to yell, and at the end of a lecture, says that the girl's behavior is going to lead the couple to divorce. The father sits quietly, looking helpless and sad. The daughter storms out of the room.

My question is, what moral intuitions did you experience as you read about this scene? I can tell you that I first felt strongly about care/harm: This was a damaging thing to say to a 15-year-old who had experienced the death of her mother and a turbulent remarriage of her father. Then I felt a sense of the unfairness to put responsibility for a divorce on the girl's shoulders (or anyone else's shoulders): Divorcing or remaining married is the responsibility of the married partners. A third intuition was about loyalty/betrayal: The father should not let his wife do this kind of thing to his children. (This was not the first or last verbal blast that his frustrated wife delivered to her stepkids.)

I invite you to focus on your moral intuitions here, as opposed to other intuitions such as diagnostic ones (does the stepmother have a personality

---

[1]The case examples in this chapter have been modified to disguise the identities of the clients involved and to protect their confidentiality.

disorder, or is the father demonstrating passive dependency?) or family systems intuitions such as dysfunctional family triangles. Although these clinical intuitions issues may be important, if we don't also process our moral and ethical intuitions, I believe we will miss something at the heart of this scenario: The girl felt unfairly harmed by her stepmother and then betrayed by her father.

I heard this story years after the event when I saw the adult daughter and her father for a therapy session aimed at healing a divide between them after the father and stepmother divorced. There was a lot to deal with in traditional clinical terms, but my willingness to access my ethical intuitions and put them into the clinical framework I've presented in this book helped to create a breakthrough at this key moment in their history: The daughter was wronged by her father and stepmother and wanted her father to acknowledge these wrongs. When he was able to do this, we could then get into the complexities of his psychological makeup (including conflict avoidance) and common patterns of remarriage and stepfamily life that they were all dealing with (e.g., setting up the new wife to be the "wicked stepmother" when the father backs away too much) and the major challenges of forming a stepfamily with teenagers. The father was able to recognize the harm he caused and how stuck he had felt between divided loyalties to his daughter and his wife. At the end of the session, the adult daughter was able to admit that she had taken out her anger toward her father on her stepmother. And she affirmed that her father and stepmother had indeed given her a good start on life, despite the problems.

Because therapists have been trained to separate the clinical and ethical domains, it's tempting to work with a case like this in strictly clinical terms. The downside is that our moral intuitions may distort our work if we don't accept them and work with them. For example, we may feel anger or even outrage at the person doing the harm or the betrayal and enact this anger by assigning diagnostic labels without enough information—or more simplistically, assume malicious motivations to the parties involved ("That woman was willing to sacrifice her stepdaughter for her own benefit").

These reactions are especially tempting when the "destructive" individual is not in the room with our client. I've heard many therapists use terms such as "flaming narcissist" or "complete borderline" or "blatant antisocial tendencies" when characterizing a spouse or family member who they see as hurting their client. The affective and the pejorative adjectives accompanying these diagnostic labels signal that the speaker is triggered by the "bad" things that someone has done. A poorly kept secret in the field is that when therapists get upset with someone (colleagues included!), we have a full quiver of personality labels to launch at them. The irony is that although we are loath to go deeply into the ethics of our clients' behavior, lest we judge and blame them, it can feel easy to do the clinical equivalent of judging and blaming people we believe are doing wrong by our clients. Unwilling to judge our clients' behavior toward others, we are quick to judge others' behavior toward our clients.

In sum, being aware of, instead of self-censoring, our moral intuitions is a key element in doing competent ethical consultation. Our moral intuitions give us clues to what our clients might be doing and experiencing. They are like any other feeling we have in the room with clients: something to consider, evaluate, and decide whether they are a reliable guide to what we do next in the therapy session.

CULTURAL SELF-AWARENESS IN ETHICAL CONSULTATION

I have argued in this book that psychotherapy is strongly influenced by its origins in Western individualist culture. In the same way, the field of medicine comes out of a Western scientific and mechanistic tradition with an emphasis on finding the smallest biological factors that cause disease—the physician becomes an applied biologist (Engel, 1977). Having an implicit cultural paradigm is not a flaw of either medicine or psychotherapy, but a lack of awareness of one's "professional culture of origin" can create blind spots and missteps. When it comes to ethical self-awareness, moral foundations theory proposes both cultural universality and cultural specificity. In other words, the five foundations of intuitive ethics are used universally across cultures but are applied differently in different environments. For example, every culture has notions of care/harm that are available to individuals when they process ethical situations. Culturally unique moralities are built on top of these intuitive foundations. Respect for elders often looks quite different around the world, even though some notion of authority and tradition is universal. Every modern culture has the moral foundation of fairness/cheating that is available to individuals contemplating decisions on paying taxes, but cultures differ on whether cheating on taxes is ethically acceptable.

As discussed in Chapter 1, Haidt (2012) found that American liberals and conservatives occupy somewhat different moral and political cultures. If we assume as likely that the majority of therapists are on the liberal side of the political spectrum, we would tend to trust care/harm and fairness/cheating as the fundamental moral intuitions while being more wary of authority, loyalty, and purity. The latter three reflect a more collectivist view of human beings that gives moral weight to authoritative institutions and traditions. If this analysis is correct, it's important for therapists to be aware of their cultural predisposition, reinforced in training, toward not recognizing the legitimacy, for some clients, of the moral sensibilities such as respect for authority, group loyalty, and avoiding impurity in thoughts and deeds. I call this a form of cultural self-awareness for the therapist, akin to recognizing the importance of one's racial and ethnic origins and influences.

I once had a memorable argument with a therapist colleague about respect for authority. I can't remember how we got into the discussion, but the upshot was that she disagreed vehemently with my notion that there was a qualitative difference between a schoolkid saying some version of "F—k off" to an annoying classmate versus saying it to the teacher. My colleague's position was that disrespect is the same negative thing regardless of the status of the one being disrespected. I asked if the same would apply to saying something disrespectful to one's sibling versus one's grandmother. No difference, she replied. I'm sure my colleague understood that the consequence to the child would be greater from disrespect to an authority figure or family elder, but in terms of moral foundations theory, she did not accept the legitimacy of authority/subversion as merit for considering the ethics of personal actions.

At the time, I didn't have Haidt's language to understand our disagreement, but now I believe my colleague was doing an ethical "override" of a universal intuition that she probably had herself, one that has been important to keep societies and families functioning. When a member of Congress shouted, "You lie!" during President Obama's 2009 State of the Union speech, this was more ethically disturbing than if he had said this to a fellow member of Congress during a heated committee debate. Although some partisans likely did an override of their intuition about showing basic respect for leaders at solemn moments, I think many Americans felt an ethical pang.

To be clear, I am not suggesting that respect for figures of authority is more important than working for fairness and justice, nor that civility toward them is a universal ethical mandate. (Some highly ethical Germans tried to assassinate Hitler.) I am saying that when therapists dismiss ethical frames unless they reflect individualist cultural norms, they are acting out of a cultural blind spot. A personal example: I recall being incredulous when a fellow graduate student from the Baha'i faith felt he needed to get permission from his parents to marry his girlfriend. I saw this as a lack of self-differentiation from his family of origin, and if he had been my client, I probably would have been unable to affirm any aspect of his moral intuition that it was important to ask elders to weigh in on this decision. (By the way, he knew they would say "yes.")

The same blind spot can occur when clients considering divorce bring up considerations such as "I made a vow when I got married" or "A divorce would affect both of our extended families." The first relates to faithfulness and loyalty, which can be in tension with current unhappiness and relationship distress. The second extends the orbit of concern beyond children to the wider kin network, a somewhat foreign idea in an individualist culture. Again, I want to be clear that I am not suggesting that these considerations ought to override other factors in a divorce decision. It's just that when clients introduce these ethical considerations, therapists are wise to accept their legitimacy for the clients rather than "help" the client see them as not useful or even unhealthy.

In my teaching and supervision with therapists of color, I've sometimes witnessed this tension between their more collectivist cultural orientation toward ethical responsibilities and the more individualistic orientation that they absorb in graduate education and clinical training. An example of how this can play out clinically for students of color is when they accept how a client makes personal sacrifices (like losing a job) when an extended family member needs their help, whereas the clinical supervisor questions these choices as self-sabotaging without acknowledging the tension between self-interest and loyalty to kin.

THE RELATIONAL, COMMITTED SELF OF THE THERAPIST

As I argued in earlier chapters, in this psychological era of history, when the interior life is explored and celebrated, therapists have shaped the image of the self for the wider culture (Rieff, 1966). I argued for a cultural shift toward the relational, committed self. Here, I connect this idea to the self of the therapist. I suggest that doing ethical consultation well requires that therapists embrace two core ideas for their own lives: that each of us as a self is (a) inherently relational and (b) defined in part by the commitments we make and keep. In other words, we are embedded in relationships that call us to faithfulness, some of them because we chose the relationship (marriage or deep friendship) and some of them because we were born and adopted into them (such as family) or find ourselves as citizens of them (our community, nation, or world). Commitment, as I wrote in Chapter 3, involves sustained investments in something outside oneself, to relationships and causes that transcend us, extend us, challenge us, and require continual struggle to manage and sometimes sacrifice for (Taylor, 1992). This is a long way from the image of the self via Fritz Perls (1969): "I do my thing, and you do your thing" (p. 4).

I have little doubt that therapists see themselves as relational beings. Indeed, our work involves developing and sustaining relationships with clients, some of whom struggle with relationship competency. Most therapists I have known are not loners: They are embedded in a number of important relationships. It's the commitment part of the relational self that I am less confident in for therapists. I wonder about therapists who seem too eager to encourage divorce during individual therapy with a client or appear too ready to encourage family cutoffs when these relationships are stressful. This seems more than a lapse in skill or allegiance to a particular model of therapy. What would lead a therapist to do what a colleague told me happened at the end of her first and only couples therapy session with her now ex-husband? At the end of the intake session, the therapist said words like these: "I've done this work for a long time, and I can pretty much tell which couples can't make it. I'm afraid you two are in that category." Ten years later and in a good second marriage, my colleague still felt shocked and abandoned by those words from the therapist, which her husband took to heart and moved immediately to divorce her, without ever explaining his reasons beyond being unhappy. I can't help but think that the ethical self of the therapist was involved here.

In addition to being influenced by a cultural norm where relationships are transactional and not permanent, there is one piece of indirect evidence that therapists may struggle with commitment in their own lives. It relates to divorce. As a backdrop, one would expect therapists to have lower than average divorce rates because of two major factors: (a) They are highly educated relative to the rest of the population, and more education nowadays is associated with considerably lower divorce rates (Amato, 2010; Copen et al., 2012); and (b) they presumably have higher than average interpersonal skills, which one would expect to make for better marriages or at least more ability to work through relational problems. That's why it's noteworthy that a large, definitive study of divorce rates among occupations, using U.S. Census data, found that the category of "therapists" showed a divorce rate 48% higher than the national average (McCoy & Aamodt, 2010). Other similar occupational categories showed the same pattern: Counselors were 38% higher than average, psychologists (some of whom are not therapists) 18%, and social workers (again, some are not therapists) 42%. This is not a matter of elevated divorce rates for all helping or highly educated professionals: Physicians were 44% below the national average, and postsecondary teachers were 15% below average.

Of course, there are a number of ways to interpret higher divorce rates among therapists other than that they have personal issues with commitment. Perhaps they have less sense of stigma about divorce and view it as a healthy alternative to a dissatisfying marriage. Perhaps their expectations are higher for marriage, and they are less willing to settle for lower quality marriages. Those may well be factors. However, both can be viewed as connected to commitment, with lower stigma making divorce a more permissible alternative and with higher expectations offsetting other constraints to remaining committed. In other words, if I expect more out of a marriage, I am more likely to be disappointed than if I expect less. And if divorce carries less shame, I am more likely to leave when my expectations are not met. All of these explanations assume that the therapist in the couple is the one initiating the divorce; perhaps their spouses (presumably, most of them nontherapists) are more likely to leave the marriage.

Whatever the explanations for higher divorce rates among therapists, we are left with the anomaly: that the profession most entrusted with helping people have good relationships has a higher level of divorce, much higher than their demographic factors would predict. How this might influence their therapy with clients considering divorce or family cutoffs is unknown. I raise the issue here because I am concerned that the combination of unacknowledged cultural norms favoring impermanence in relationships and personal experience with divorce could lead therapists to undervalue the ethic of commitment and unknowingly encourage unnecessary or premature divorces.

ETHICAL CARING BEYOND OUR CLIENTS

Caring for our clients is in the soul of therapy. Clients have to know that we understand them, accept them, are invested in them as unique persons, and want to promote their well-being. We have no medications or surgical techniques that work well regardless of our attitude toward our clients. It's us and them in a relationship of trust. Here, I want to argue that caring for our clients also means caring for the people whose lives they touch, something that's hard to do when those people are at odds with our clients.

The philosopher Nel Noddings (1984) made a helpful distinction between "natural caring" and "ethical caring." *Natural caring* stems from a spontaneous desire to accept and respond to the other person, with the paradigmatic example being the caring of a parent for a child. In therapy, natural caring comes most easily for the therapist when the client is open with us about their distress and responds appreciatively to our offer of help. I suspect that natural caring comes to us readily with most of our clients.

Not so for the "difficult" client who withholds parts of the story, is ambivalent about receiving help, or complains that we are not doing enough.

Whereas natural caring involves the ability to respond spontaneously to those who entrust their pain to us, *ethical caring* is called for when we find it hard to make a caring connection with a client. We may dislike the client or be turned off by the client's behavior inside and outside the therapy room. In these situations, according to Noddings' framework, we have to call on our ethical ideal of being a caring person to access our sensitivity and responsivity to someone for whom our inclinations are not sufficient. This caring is ethical in the sense that I believe "I must" try to respond to the other. It's my duty as a therapist. Noddings proposed that when blocked from natural caring, we can call on our experiences of being cared for as children and throughout our lives. These experiences and memories give us the strength "to strive to meet the other morally" (p. 10).

Here I want to extend Noddings's concept of ethical caring to how we think about other people in our clients' lives. If the ethical domain in therapy is how we address the consequences of our clients' decisions and actions for the welfare of others, then the needs and experiences of those others are inevitably present in our work. We are always affecting people who are in the client's life but not in the room with us. We can either see them as not our responsibility or as "clients once removed." I'm in the latter camp, partly because of my background in family therapy and partly because of my investment in the ethical domain of therapy.

This book has many examples of the negative consequences when therapists ignore the potential effects of client behavior for other people. But sometimes, it's the therapist who initiates a process that can lead to harmful outcomes for third parties. I recall a famous therapist recounting a case where she coached a shy man who was afraid of women in how to get dates by telling women that he was interested in a serious relationship when, in fact, he was simply trying to develop his dating skills. It worked for him, she said. I remember sitting in that seminar feeling uncomfortable that this brilliant therapist was not concerned about the women her client was deceiving (not to mention the compromise to the client's integrity). I found myself wondering whether anyone else in the room felt as I did. I wish I had spoken up or at least asked the therapist about it later.

Then there is the issue of how therapists talk about the important people in their clients' lives. I haven't kept track of all the times that clients have told me that their individual therapist offered a diagnosis of the client's spouse, usually with a personality disorder, thereby confirming the client's sense that their spouse was the dysfunctional one and that there was no changing them. (All this without the therapist having met the spouse.) This kind of intervention violates professional ethics, and it's a lapse of ethical caring because it labels and objectifies someone central in the client's life.

TABLE 7.1. Individual Therapy Clients Report on Therapist Diagnosis of Spouse's/Partner's Mental Health (*n* = 101)

Item: My counselor suggested that my spouse/partner had a personality or mental health diagnosis without having done an individual assessment.

Response	Frequency	%	Cumulative %
1 Not at all true	45	44.6	44.6
2 Somewhat true	13	12.9	57.4
3 Moderately true	18	17.8	75.2
4 Mostly true	10	9.9	85.1
5 Completely true	14	13.9	99.0
6 Don't know/can't remember	1	1.0	100.0
Total	101	100.0	

After years of complaining about this phenomenon, which makes my work as a couples therapist more difficult, I decided to gather data to document the phenomenon and see how widespread it is. For research submitted for publication, my colleagues Steve Harris, Eugene Hall, and I surveyed 101 individuals who had brought relationship issues to individual therapy. It was a national sample gathered from Mturk, an online platform often used by social scientists to gather samples that, while not nationally representative, are superior to most other kinds of convenience samples. Here, I describe participant responses when asked whether their therapist had made two kinds of statements: (a) "My counselor suggested that my spouse/partner had a personality or mental health diagnosis without having done an individual assessment," and (b) "Without ever having met my spouse/partner, my counselor suggested that my spouse/partner was unlikely to change." The Likert response scale ranged from *not true at all* to *completely true*. Tables 7.1 and 7.2 present the results.

TABLE 7.2. Individual Therapy Clients Report on Therapist Statements Regarding Spouse's/Partner's Unlikeliness to Change (*n* = 101)

Item: Without ever having met my spouse/partner, my counselor suggested that my spouse/partner was unlikely to change.

Response	Frequency	%	Cumulative %
1 Not at all true	36	35.6	35.6
2 Somewhat true	18	17.8	53.5
3 Moderately true	16	15.8	69.3
4 Mostly true	18	17.8	87.1
5 Completely true	11	10.9	98.0
6 Don't know/can't remember	2	2.0	100.0
Total	101	100.0	

For interpreting the findings, my colleagues and I proposed that ethically responsible practice by the therapist should be represented by *not true at all*. With that guideline, over half of clients reported that their therapist said these things (53% for diagnosing the spouse and 64% for suggesting that the spouse could not change). If we loosen the guideline to allow for *somewhat true*, the numbers are still sobering (43% and 46%, respectively), as they are if we extend the limit to the categories of *mostly true* or *completely true* (23% and 28%, respectively). Of course, it's not possible to know whether the clients heard their therapist correctly or remembered accurately. However, the findings do suggest that these therapist actions are not rare. They are a troubling indicator of the absence of a sense of responsibility for the consequences of our statements for our clients' relationships and their intimate partners.

I'll state my position bluntly: We have an ethical responsibility to care about the welfare of people whose lives intersect with the lives of our clients. At a minimum, this means not doing something to harm them, which includes not diagnosing them without directly assessing them and not pronouncing them incapable of change (something a therapist has no way of knowing for sure). And beyond that, it means holding mental images of these third parties as complex persons with their own goals and aspirations, as opposed to being cardboard characters or minor, disposable characters in the theater of our clients' lives.

I once had a teacher who tried to ease our newbie-therapist anxieties by saying that it's at least as hard to really harm a client as it is to really help them. I was comforted at the time, but I eventually stopped believing it. Maybe it's true for routine moments of therapy, but at times of ethical intensity in our clients' lives, we have the power to help or harm them in equal measure. That's why being attuned to our ethical, caring, and relational self is essential at every moment in every session, for the sake of our clients and the social ecology around them.

This leads to the final chapter on the larger role of the therapist in society.

8 THE CITIZEN THERAPIST

When I was a graduate student in the 1970s, I imagined that if we could get all members of Congress into a good marathon encounter group, government reform and social justice would not be far behind. Underneath this naive idea was a kind of "trickle-up" assumption that if we therapists made enough people psychologically healthy, then by a kind of osmosis, the social order would become healthy and fair for everyone. Years later, I came across a book titled *We've Had a Hundred Years of Psychotherapy—And the World's Getting Worse*. Written in the 1990s by noted Jungian therapist James Hillman and writer James Ventura (Hillman & Ventura, 1993), its title and message resonate in the 2020s.

When I was writing *Soul Searching* in the early 1990s, therapists were beginning to address in earnest the toxic influences of broad societal issues, such as racism and sexism, on our clients. By the third decade of the 21st century, the literature on the role of societal oppression on clients is rich and deep, covering additional domains such as the antigay, antitrans effects on clients and the benefits of taking an "intersectional" approach that can encompass the effects on people who have more than one marginalized social status (e.g., being Black and gay). For therapists who want to increase

https://doi.org/10.1037/0000263-009

their sensitivity and skills in addressing societal forces affecting clients with identities outside of mainstream, heterosexual White America, there are rich resources available. Examples of this literature include Aldarondo (2008), Comas-Díaz (2020), and Lee (2018).

In this chapter, I want to fill in three gaps I see in current work on socially just therapy. First is the implicit assumption that societal forces only come into play when treating clients in a minority group—sexual, racial, and others. In my view, toxic social forces can affect everyone who comes to therapy, even straight, upper-middle-class White men. Second is an imbalance in the literature, which focuses on how clients experience and cope with oppressive social forces, with too little attention to how they can be agents of change in their communities. Third is an assumption that therapists' role in social justice work occurs almost exclusively in the therapy office, not in the community.

THERAPISTS AND SOCIAL CHANGE

First, let's back up to why it's been hard to conceptualize the role of the therapist in social change. As I discussed in the Introduction and Chapter 1, the field was created to help individuals cope with their psychological problems and later, through couples therapy and family therapy, with their current relational problems. The client's place in the larger world was mostly invisible, and beyond that, there was a tendency to be skeptical of clients' commitments to the larger world. I brought this up once at a writers retreat during a presentation to fellow writers. I referred to a bias of traditional therapy toward the inner world and a tendency to see work for the public good as stemming from unmet inner needs. During the subsequent discussion, a married couple spoke up about their experience in therapy.[1] Their work involved going to towns in the northwestern United States that were facing environmental challenges with the logging industry. They helped local community members organize and find their voices through making public art. The work was funded by a series of small grants, giving the couple little financial stability. They were at the writers retreat working on a book to make their work more visible and spread its reach.

I'll never forget the dismay this couple expressed after they heard my presentation. They said they had each been in and out of individual therapy for years, and in fact, many of their friends in the Bay Area of California were

---

[1]The case examples in this chapter have been modified to disguise the identities of the clients involved and to protect their confidentiality.

therapists. From their own therapists, they experienced more challenge than support for their civic work—for example, questions about what unmet psychological needs were leading them to try to save the world. And from their therapist friends, they reported ongoing teasing about when they were going to grow up and get real jobs. Until hearing that this feedback represented a bias in the therapy field, they had felt discomfited by the feedback but did not question it. Now they were angry.

Several years later, at a conference, I heard a case description in which the client was reported to be burned out by her work with homeless and other needy people in her city. She was overworking and not paying attention to her personal needs. The therapist described her repeated efforts to help her client see that she was trying to make up for unmet needs from her family of origin and ruining her health in the process. I had no problem with the case description thus far—there can be multiple reasons why anyone loses their life balance in service to others. But then came the clincher. After reporting that the client did indeed quit her job, the therapist noted, "I was not able to her get to completely stop being a world saver: She ended up as a manager in another small nonprofit in the inner city." I was stunned as I asked myself, "What would complete success have looked like—the client taking a job as a hedge fund manager?"

A final example: A therapist colleague who had worked on international population issues for decades confessed to me, after hearing my critique of the private-world bias of psychotherapy, that she suddenly realized that at times of her life when she was not in personal therapy, she was making her contributions to population control, whereas when she would go back to therapy, she would be encouraged by her therapist to focus only on her inner world. The message she got was that her "outer world" efforts were a way to avoid the personal work she needed to do. Like the woman serving the homeless, the therapy did not help integrate her inner world with her ethical commitment to the public good.

In sum, I am arguing that the blind spots of traditional psychotherapy include the civic lives of the people who seek our help. To address this domain will require pushing the conceptual boundaries of moral foundations theory (Haidt & Joseph, 2007), described in Chapter 1. The five moral foundations (care/harm, fairness/cheating, etc.) in this model apply more readily to the microsocial world—our moral intuitions about how we treat individuals and groups—than to the civic or public world. Here I am following the work of Janoff-Bulman and Carnes (2018), who noted that moral foundations theory does not have a clear way to conceptualize the social order and social justice—morality at the collective level. These authors made a distinction between two areas of collective ethical intuitions: caring about *social order* (how society holds together by regulating behavior—think traffic laws) and *social justice* (how society promotes sharing, equality, and communal responsibility—think affirmative action). According to Janoff-Bulman and Carnes, the first is a more prominent moral intuition for conservatives and the second for liberals. I find these ideas useful for thinking about the civic lives of clients and therapists alike. Ethics and morality are not just personal and familial—they are collective. But thinking this way in therapy involves an expansion of the image of the therapist beyond that of healer of the mind or intimate relationships.

WHAT IS A CITIZEN THERAPIST?

Much of my work in the past 25 years has been to develop the idea of the "citizen therapist" in theory and action (Doherty, 2008, 2020b; Doherty et al., 2010). There are two fundamental axioms for being a model citizen therapist:

- All clinical problems have public dimensions.
- Human beings influence larger social and environmental forces that, in turn, influence them.

In the first axiom, "public" means social, cultural, economic, environmental, and institutional influences. These larger forces are sometimes implicated in what causes clinical problems, and they are always part of the meaning making and coping with clinical problems. I believe there are no exceptions to this axiom: There are no problems we see in therapy that are without broader connections and influences. Depression, anxiety, personality disorders, psychotic disorders, and marital problems all occur in a matrix of social and environmental forces. It's just that we tend to keep those in the background as we do our clinical work.

The second axiom refers to the bidirectional influence that humans and their environments have on each other. Through individual and collective actions, we develop our social world and influence the natural world. This means that individually we have some role, even if minor in many situations, in shaping that world that shapes us. There are two implications of this bidirectional path of influence. First, psychotherapy can help people increase their capacity to contribute as members of wider communities. In other words, clinical conversations can fruitfully integrate the personal and public dimensions of people's lives. Second, the therapist can play a direct role in the public domain, working to influence the social forces that show up in the therapy room.

Wrapping these ideas together is the role of the citizen therapist in a democracy: understanding and working with the personal and public worlds of clients and being willing to engage directly in promoting the health of communities and the larger world.

THE CITIZEN THERAPIST IN THE OFFICE

I want to introduce the term *public stress* as an overarching concept for what many clients bring to therapy. It refers to how neighborhood, community, cultural, medical, employment, historical, religious, economic, political, legal, institutional, and environmental factors create challenges for personal and relational well-being (Doherty, 2017b). In terms of Bronfenbrenner's (1979) ecological model, these influences can range from micro to macro systems. One type of public stress can be termed *political stress*, referring to how the words, actions, and policies of government bodies, elected officials, candidates for public office, and our fellow citizens create challenges for personal and relational well-being. Embracing the concept of public stress can help therapists expand our purview beyond the intrapsychic and intimate spheres in a way that feels connected to our mission as healers. In other words, the public and political forces get named along with the personal stress they are causing in the lives of clients.

Two events of the year 2020 brought all of this to the forefront for many therapists and clients alike: the COVID-19 pandemic and the presidential election. Caseloads and case consultations were suffused with discussions of how the pandemic exacerbated psychological and interpersonal issues for clients and therapists alike. Adding to this historic level of public stress, where public health becomes as important as medical care, was tension from a historically polarized political election season. Not only were politicians battling each other but family members and friends were also staking out sides against one another (Finkel et al., 2020). Politics also affected public health through the division of opinions about wearing face masks. For therapists, there was no escaping the role of public and political forces influencing our clients' lives.

As with all professions, our intake paperwork reflects which areas of clients' lives we are interested in and which are outside of our interest. Thus, if we confine our questions to psychological symptoms, we suggest we are not very interested in the clients' interpersonal relationships. In the same way, I believe the absence of any questions about our clients' public lives sends a message. So several years ago I decided to develop two intake questions dealing with the public lives of my new clients. One question addresses public stress and the other public engagement. Here they are:

- Sometimes, people in counseling feel stress from events and forces in their community, the nation, or the world. If that's true for you, I encourage you to briefly let me know. (Otherwise, just skip this section.) Here's what's causing me stress: [list your stress-causing item(s)].

- Sometimes, people in counseling have commitments to groups or causes outside of their family and close social world. If that's true for you, briefly write what those commitments are for you. Otherwise, just leave this section blank.

Although I estimate that before the COVID-19 pandemic, only a quarter of my clients answered these items on the intake (I explicitly give them permission not to answer), I've found that these answers can open doors to my understanding what's affecting them from the larger world and what they are proud of in their community roles. During the 2020–2021 COVID-19 pandemic, more clients brought up environmental fears. Other clients expressed their political stress related to elections.

What if there is considerable political stress in the community? Is there a place for this in therapy? A therapist attuned to political stress gave a workshop for mental health professionals in Argentina, many of whom had been in practice during the horrible "disappearances," when thousands of ordinary citizens were kidnapped and murdered by government officials. The workshop leader asked the audience, "What was it like to treat patients during that time?" He was met with silence and blank stares. The issue had not come up in the mainly psychoanalytic therapy practiced at the time. It was outside the model, like the original Latin meaning of the word *obscene*: off stage.

As mentioned, there is now more permission for U.S. therapists to explore stress related to discrimination and microaggressions that clients face as individuals with minority identities. I am arguing here for allowing public stress to be part of the work with all clients, including those considered privileged in mainstream society. For example, I have explored with middle-class parents the pressure they feel to provide enrichment experiences for their children in a competitive culture, even though they end up compromising the quality of family time and family life (Doherty & Carlson, 2003). Early in my career, I would have ignored the cultural pressures and focused only on my clients' feelings and decisions about what to do for their child. Now I am also willing to discuss the toxic cultural forces that they and their peers are facing. If we don't attend to cultural forces such as the anxious, hypercompetitive culture of parenting, we will overemphasize intrapsychic issues—for example, seeing personal fantasies or insecurities driving the client's parenting. Stated differently, when the model community member is behaving in what seems to be a dysregulated way, look first at cultural factors and then at individual factors.

Once clients open up about their public and political stress, we have a variety of therapeutic tools to help them. Some of these are stress-buffering methods such as self-care, cutting back on time spent on news coverage and social media, and not letting yourself get baited by the political gladiators in your life. Other stress management methods involve active coping with public and political stress. They might take steps to become better informed about public issues. Clients might donate to political leaders they respect or to nonprofits making the world better. They could get directly involved in a political campaign or a public protest. On an everyday level, they can reach out personally to neighbors who might be feeling stress about how their ethnic or racial group is being treated.

We can also help clients process emotionally dysregulated reactions to public officials or environmental events. Colleagues have told me that the COVID-19 pandemic has brought out old traumas that clients had not previously disclosed in therapy. And bullying by political officials can activate feelings of having been mistreated as children. Outer and inner worlds interact for all of us as social being.

In dealing with political stress in particular, our job is to help clients find a grounded/responsive stance rather than two less functional alternatives: numb/reactive (akin to the "freeze" response) or agitated/reactive (highly aroused and preoccupied). Being grounded and responsive is where we can identify and accept our feelings and make choices about how to act according to our values. In family relationships, this means being able to live with sharp political differences without having to change the other person or becoming cut off from that person (Safer, 2019). Therapy with a public dimension can be an incubator for connected and empowered citizenship.

Next, I address specific strategies for allowing public stress into therapy and sometimes initiating conversations about it.

HOW TO BRING UP PUBLIC STRESS IN THERAPY

Because therapists and clients alike have been socialized into a personal and public split, with therapy being only about the personal domain, it's not automatic that clients will bring up the stress they are feeling about today's political environment. So, it's up to us to be intentional and skillful about creating a space for these conversations. The following are three ways that clients can bring up public issues in therapy sessions and three ways that therapists can bring them up.

How Clients Bring Up a Public Issue

Sometimes, clients bring up public or political stress obliquely at the beginning of a session—for example, in an offhanded comment, while settling into the session, about the latest thing that a political leader has done or said. You can take these "side comments" seriously and ask clients how they are feeling about what's going on with the political scene. If the client seems eager to talk, the therapist can either keep the topic going or be more explicit by saying something such as, "We can spend a bit of time on this if you like, or we can move on to other matters."

Second, in the middle of a session, a client may compare a personal concern with a public one—for example, by saying that a relative reminds them of a political leader and then perhaps laughing, as if to suggest that it was strange to bring a public figure into the therapy conversation, or by mentioning a desire to avoid political conflict with relatives at an upcoming gathering. You can say, "That sounds like something to dig into a little. How is your relative like [the public figure] in your life?" or "How are you and your family member divided by politics?"

The third way is more direct: The client brings up personal stress connected to a public figure or issue. The citizen therapist's task here is not only to acknowledge this at the personal level (individual stress and coping) but also to invite conversation about how the client's political and civic values are involved.

How Therapists Can Bring Up a Public Issue

Public issues are new territory for most therapists and require judgment calls about which clients and at what time it might help to initiate the conversation. One approach is to open a session with a query about whether the client has any thoughts or concerns about what's going on in this divided world these days. During a presidential campaign, for example, I sometimes have asked clients whether they were following the campaign and, if so, whether it was creating any stress for them.

A second approach is to note a major community or national event, preferably during the initial getting-settled phase of the session. These events would normally be public knowledge through the news media or a topic of local community conversation—for example, "Are the local policing protests affecting you or your home or work situations?"

The third approach may occur during the session when a client is talking about unusual levels of emotional stress or physical discomfort (one client talked about the return of her "eyelid twitch," a sign she is under stress). The therapist can ask whether the client sees any connection with what's going on in the larger political world that is upsetting to a lot of people.

The idea here is not to treat the therapy room as if it's a bubble cut off from events that we have reason to think are affecting our clients. Surfacing a public or political issue is often all that happens in a session: briefly noted as something of concern or no particular concern at the moment. The client often moves directly on to other material in the session or sometimes lingers and wants to delve into these concerns. Either way, what has happened is an implicit understanding in the therapy relationship that public issues have a place in the conversation between the therapist and client. The world is bigger than the personal and microsocial world generally discussed in therapy. People can bring their public selves with them instead of checking them at the door.

THE CITIZEN THERAPIST IN A DEMOCRACY[2]

The stressful elections of 2016 and 2020 helped me better see the connection between psychotherapy and democracy. Both are about the sense of agency or efficacy, especially when democracy is viewed as not only as a governmental system but as collective agency ("we the responsible people") for solving problems and building a common world. There cannot be collective efficacy without the kind of personal efficacy that therapists promote in our work, and personal efficacy is compromised in nations when democracy is compromised or not present at all. When we do our jobs well, we are developing citizens of democracies. Collective agency cannot exist without personal agency (Doherty, 2017b, 2017c).

It goes the other way too. I believe that therapy needs the larger system of democracy in order to thrive. I've trained international students who went home to dictatorial government systems that greatly inhibited what these

[2]Portions of this section are from "My Journey as a Citizen Therapist," by W. J. Doherty, 2020b, *Journal of Humanistic Psychology*, *60*(4), pp. 477–487 (https://doi.org/10.1177/0022167819899594). Copyright 2020 by Sage. Adapted with permission.

therapists could encourage their clients to say and do in their social world. One therapist had to do her group work with adolescents in the woods rather than in her office because visible group gatherings could raise the suspicions of government officials. The Argentinian therapists I mentioned may have been afraid that their clients would report them for asking about the "disappearances" or encouraging them to speak out. Empowering people to be responsible for their thoughts and actions can have repercussions for the client and the therapist alike in autocratic nations.

The same is true in a long-term democracy when leaders threaten its core institutions. A therapist working with young protestors could be exposed to public reprimands and private threats for encouraging action for social change. Researchers working on psychological "denial" about the threats of pandemics or climate change could be blackballed. These are threats from the political right. For balance, I want to point out that antidemocratic tendencies on the political left (e.g., in the form of language policing) also bring risks to the ability of therapists to practice free speech and promote client agency. Some people are driven to seek help in therapy because they crossed a political line drawn by people on the left of the political spectrum. In my view, political extremes on either side quickly become antidemocratic, by which I mean they oppose personal and collective agency if it does not fit their parameters for speech and behavior.

My conclusion is that to fulfill the potential of our professional role in a democracy, we have to be active outside our offices to counteract forces that bring clients to our offices or complicate their lives. I've been involved in a number of public projects using the families and democracy model and citizen health care models that I developed with Tai Mendenhall and Jerica Berge (Doherty, 2020b; Doherty et al., 2010). Here, I focus on two projects close to my heart on key issues of our time: political polarization and racial justice.

A Therapist Works on Political Depolarization

Although I had been involved in public engagement work for many years, I did not step into the arena of political conflict and polarization until I was galvanized by a 2016 trip to Austria, which was in the midst of a presidential election campaign featuring an explicitly neofascist candidate. I observed brown-shirted neofascist youth convening in a small town to support their candidate. I then read about the silence of mental health professionals during the rise of national socialism in Germany in the 1930s.

This experience confirmed my sense that U.S. presidential candidate Donald Trump was a danger beyond policies or personality but to American democracy itself. I decided to try to mobilize my fellow therapists by writing a manifesto called "Citizen Therapists Against Trumpism," which attracted over 2,500 signatures, among which were those of prominent leaders in the therapy world. What followed were media interviews where I articulated my concerns as a therapist that Trumpism and the Trump presidency were a threat to our democracy. For the first time, I embraced the connection between democracy as "collective agency" (we the people building a common life and solving problems together) and the everyday practice of therapy in promoting personal agency or efficacy. Therapy, I concluded, is considered a form of democratic practice (Doherty, 2017b, 2017c). There is no democracy unless individuals and families have the kind of agency that authoritarian, antidemocratic regimes seek to undermine.

After the election of Donald Trump, I shifted to a different kind of democratic work: to reduce the toxic polarization rising in the country. The backdrop is the rise over several decades of social (or affective) polarization where ordinary Americans have come to regard people who vote differently as untrustworthy enemies (Finkel et al., 2020; Hetherington & Weiler, 2018; Mason, 2018). I sensed that the battle against Trumpism would attract many advocates, whereas the effort to bridge the bitter partisan divide (which contributed to the rise of Trumpism) needed dedicated staffers. I assumed at first that I would do this work by organizing therapists to promote psychotherapy as a democratic practice in a pluralistic but divided world. Then a surprise invitation sent me in a different direction.

Braver Angels

About 10 days after the 2016 election, I received a phone call from my colleague David Blankenhorn, with whom I had worked on a project bringing together gay marriage advocates and religious liberty advocates to search for understanding and common ground on that contentious issue. For that work, I had called on the group process training I had as a graduate student and continued to use in my career. David told me that when he talked with our mutual colleague David Lapp shortly after the election, they saw a stark contrast: Blankenhorn's Manhattan neighborhood was in shock and grief after the election, while Lapp's community in Southwest Ohio was practically dancing in the streets. They realized that if there was ever a time to go bold on polarization, this was it. So, they decided to invite 10 Hillary Clinton and

10 Donald Trump supporters from Southwest Ohio to spend 13 hours over a weekend to see whether they could meet each other as concerned Americans and not as enemies. I knew I had to sign on to help design and facilitate the gathering (see Doherty, 2017a).

That weekend of December 9–11, 2016, was a big success—people met each other across their differences. I left with the belief that most Democrats and Republicans do not want a civic divorce and, if offered the right structure and process for conversation, will choose to listen and eventually find common ground. My check-out words at the end were, "This weekend I've felt the pain of our nation, and now I feel hope for our nation."

Out of that weekend workshop in 2016 came the national nonprofit Better Angels (later renamed Braver Angels after a trademark dispute; Better Angels was from the Abraham Lincoln phrase "the better angels of our nature"). The mission is to bring conservatives and liberals (reds and blues) together to depolarize America. The main vehicle is workshops that help people move beyond stereotypes to find common ground and train people in constructive ways to discuss political differences. In addition to the flagship "red–blue" workshop (a 3- or 7-hour experience with equal numbers of reds and blues), I also developed workshops on Skills for Bridging the Divide, on Depolarizing Within, where people learn to change their hearts and minds and serve as agents of depolarization within their political communities, and on Families and Politics, where people learn how to relate to family members who differ politically. April Lawson, a Braver Angels colleague, developed a special debate process that encourages a collective search for understanding rather than winning or losing, and Reena Bernards, a therapist and Braver Angels colleague, developed a Common Ground workshop on specific issues such as abortion and climate change. We've trained several hundred workshop moderators who have led workshops across the country (over a thousand workshops by January 2021). All moderator training is free, and all workshops are free. After participating in a workshop, people are invited to join local Braver Angels Alliances groups. And I'm glad to report that local and national public officials are reaching out to work with Braver Angels.

A key policy decision made early in the development of Braver Angels was that every level of leadership will consist of equal numbers of reds and blues (plus people who do not identify as red or blue). This policy gives Braver Angels a degree of credibility, especially with conservatives who tend to be skeptical about what they see as the liberal bent of groups who work on intergroup conflict (as well as the psychological professions in general). I have experienced great value in these cross-political relationships, which have made me "bilingual" in today's divided world—I can speak red or blue.

Here is the connection to therapy. As a couples therapist, I am used to dealing with polarized people. Success depends first on connecting with both partners. In the same way, I cannot be helpful as a citizen therapist unless I can understand and speak the languages of both sides of the political divide. Of course, this can be more than with couples (whose relationship I am not a part of) because I am an insider when it comes to political divides: I have my own strong values and views on who should win elections and lead the country. But in other ways, it's a similar process: how to bring divided people together across differences to solve problems—in the case of the country, how to form "a more perfect union" in a multipartisan and multiracial democracy that is struggling. This means accessing what couples have to find: what glues us together, what we care about in common, and what we want for ourselves and our offspring, both personally and collectively. And it requires in the political domain what couples come to see in successful therapy: that they both contributed to the polarization and stalemate, and each can contribute to the movement forward. That humility factor—offering opportunities to look in the mirror and not just point fingers—is a key element from couples therapy that I carried over into the work of Braver Angels.

The Police and Black Men Project

My hometown of Minneapolis has become the epicenter of problems between police and the Black community. This project came out of a 2016 conversation with my colleague Guy Bowling when the local community was devastated by the unnecessary police killing of Philando Castile after a traffic stop a mile from my home. Guy told me that he was reaching "outrage fatigue" as a Black man and asked whether the families and democracy model he and I had worked with (Doherty et al., 2010) could be applied to the problems between Minneapolis police and Black men. We then cooked up the idea that a small group of police officers and Black men would go deep to develop relationships of trust to bridge that divide.

After many conversations with police leaders, a group of five police officers (three White and two Black) and six Black men from the community began biweekly meetings in January 2017, with the mission of forging connections between police officers and African American men that can lead to better partnerships for community safety and law enforcement. Using a process I designed and facilitated, we began with rounds of storytelling (early experiences with police officers, Black men, and White men), then opened up challenging topics, such as local and national police shootings of unarmed Black men. We eventually created a common narrative document to describe who we are, how we see the problem, and the changes we envision. The group developed a remarkable level of trust and vulnerability, with men from each side talking about their pain and trauma, receiving support from everyone in the room.

The Police and Black Men Project (www.policeandblackmen.org) went public in fall 2018 with community conversations, police training, and advocacy for systemic changes beginning with safe, affordable housing. The housing issue emerged as a priority because the group realized that poor housing opportunities create unsafe conditions for both community members and police who are asked to evict people. The group's narrative statement articulates the sources of distrust between police and the Black community, the beliefs we hold in common, a vision for safe communities, and a paradigm of shared partnership for community safety. It offers a critique of prevailing paradigms that emphasize police accountability only (the liberal paradigm) or personal responsibility only (the conservative paradigm). We want to move the public conversation beyond finger pointing to one of partnership for the ultimate goal that both sides embrace: safe communities that are good places for citizens and police officers alike.

For me, the Police and Black Men Project has been an experience in the power of taking time to build relationships. As noted, we began with storytelling. In those stories, we talked about our fathers. We then moved into more conflictual conversations, with everyone committed to returning to the table over and over, no matter what, because the stakes were so high. This bond of trust, even brotherhood, was necessary for the extremely painful conversation after George Floyd's killing. First, the community members vented their anger, fear, and despair. The officers listened and condemned what their fellow officers had done. Two weeks later, the community members were there to support the officers, who were experiencing ridicule and abuse, particularly from White progressives in the community, even extending to harassment of their families. The group lost one of its police members who quit the Minneapolis Police Department to work elsewhere, but the group has survived a world-shaking event in George Floyd's killing and is making plans for the next phase of this difficult but necessary work.

An impact of this project on me can be seen on my front lawn, where I have two signs: one with the words "Black Lives Matter" and one with the words "We Care About Police Officers." Just as I can't help a couple unless I care about and advocate for both people, it's the same for police and Black people in communities. This does not mean that I see both sides as having equal responsibility for the problems—that's often not true with couples or police–community relations where the professionals carry more responsibility for historical abuses of power that have led to so much mistrust. But I do believe that both sides have to be part of solutions, with humility and courage.

HOW TO GET STARTED IN THE PUBLIC ROLE AS A CITIZEN THERAPIST

I realize that my examples of public engagement may feel beyond the immediate reach of many readers; indeed, they came after more than 2 decades of community work when the right opportunities arose. Here are some ways I recommend to begin public engagement work for those who are interested:

- **Identify your clinical passion and connect it to the larger picture.** If you are interested in trauma, look for where it is showing up in people's lives in your community. Read up on the public health dimensions of trauma in addition to the clinical dimensions.

- **Connect to a community.** This next step is pivotal: find a community to work with outside your professional world. This isn't as hard as it sounds. Start with communities you're already connected to. It might be the neighborhood you work in, the schools your kids attend and where you've given talks to PTA groups, or your religious community. A colleague of mine connected with a local public school that was interested in trauma-informed pedagogy and school experience for kids.

- **Listen for public stories.** This can come from showing up at community gatherings, attending meetings of groups such as NAMI (National Alliance for the Mentally Ill), or spending time in Facebook groups of people dealing with a clinical issue you care about. If you give public presentations on your clinical topic, devote half the time to eliciting stories of challenges and real-world successes. That's what I did when I began my citizen professional work on the issue of overscheduled kids. Lots of the public were listening.

- **Link the personal to the communal—in public.** This is easier to do nowadays with the internet, where you can use a professional Facebook or Twitter account to communicate your messages. But there is no substitute for engaging with existing groups and communities who are concerned with the same issue you are. Either way, the theme is one of I and We—problems are not merely personal; they also belong to communities.

- **Invite recipients of services to become citizen activists.** The key to public-facing work as a citizen therapist is to engage with other citizens not as clients but as coworkers on problems. If you are only talking to professionals or giving talks to community members, you will not have the full experience of citizen therapist work. Look for organizations or Facebook communities of people who have a personal stake in your issue and pitch in to add what you know and can do in cooperation with them.

- **Be open to new issues and different communities.** Once you begin to experience the identity of citizen therapist, new opportunities will come your way, as happened with me over and over. I've learned that I don't have to be an expert in an issue to get involved, learn about it, and make my contribution. You can learn as you go.

CITIZEN THERAPISTS AND CIVIC RENEWAL

I consider the Police and Black Men Project and the Braver Angels the high points of my journey as a citizen therapist. Along with my fellow psychotherapists, I believe that people have the capacity for self-healing and positive change in their personal and relational lives. Allowing the public dimensions into the therapy room is one important frontier for psychotherapy. And the public sphere needs the beliefs, knowledge, and skills of therapists, not as experts in how people should construct their public lives but as catalysts for we-the-responsible-people to act together to solve problems and forge a new, more active citizenship. The renewal of our commonwealth will not come from electing the right politicians and hoping that they can miraculously fix things for us. We need a new breed of representatives for the public good who possess the skills and knowledge to bring people together in a world that pulls us apart. Citizen therapists are obvious candidates for the job.

Afterword

Two Therapy Cases That Had a Public Impact

A theme of this book is that therapy affects more than the clients in treatment. I close with stories of two psychotherapy cases that have impacted not only the clients but also the broader culture and the nation. These examples with high-profile clients illustrate the potential consequences of ignoring the moral challenges that come up in therapy.

THE CASE OF WOODY ALLEN

After I finished the main writing of this book, I watched a new HBO documentary on the Woody Allen/Mia Farrow legal battles of the early 1990s (Dick & Ziering, 2021). The impetus for revisiting the story was that Mia Farrow finally went public with her side of the struggle that began after the revelation of Allen's sexual relationship with her adopted child Soon-Yi. I was stunned by what Farrow reported about an exchange with Allen's therapist.

Recall that in Chapter 4, I wrote about Allen's infidelity with a young woman who was functionally his stepdaughter (even though he and Farrow never legally married). I recounted my radio exchange with a New York

https://doi.org/10.1037/0000263-010
The Ethical Lives of Clients: Transcending Self-Interest in Psychotherapy, by W. J. Doherty

psychoanalyst who said she would never raise an ethical concern with a client like Allen unless the other person involved were a minor and therefore legally protected. I quoted the judge in the custody trial, who was bewildered by the neutrality of the expert psychological witnesses. Although I imagined that Allen was in his own therapy at the time, I did not have access to what Allen's therapist thought about the situation.

In the HBO documentary, Mia Farrow told the interviewer that after she discovered nude photos of Soon-Yi in Allen's apartment and confronted him, she asked Allen whether she could talk to his therapist because she didn't believe that he was telling the therapist the truth. Allen agreed as long as he could be present. As Farrow recounted the scene, she showed the photos to the therapist and told him that she was worried for Soon-Yi and her younger children, and she was fearful of losing her relationship with Soon-Yi, whom she had adopted at age 8 after a horrendous experience of abandonment and living on the streets. Farrow pleaded with the therapist to reassure her that what Allen had done would not happen anymore, including to her younger daughter and Allen's biological child. Here is how Farrow recounted in *Allen v. Farrow* (Dick & Ziering, 2021) what was said next:

THERAPIST: It's not a therapist's job to moralize.

FARROW: Well, you have a patient with no moral compass. Then I guess he's lost because this may be a moral issue.

For me, this represents a "smoking gun" example of the ethical blind spot of traditional psychotherapy. (Although it's possible that Farrow had a distorted recollection, I am inclined to accept her recounting of the conversation in part because it was so startling to her—most members of the public would not expect a therapist to define the therapist role in this way.) Note that the therapist used the term "moralize," as if his only options were to stay away from morality altogether or lecture and shame the client (i.e., moralize). I wrote this book to offer a third way.

Woody Allen had a long history with psychotherapy, particularly psychoanalysis, and spoke about it often. (See a famous interview with Dick Cavett; cavettbiter, 2007.) In the scenario described by Farrow, we see a therapist claiming that his office was a moral-free zone and a client who had once written this classic movie line about morality: "Guilt is petit-bourgeois crap. An artist creates his own moral universe" (Allen, 1994). No wonder Allen was willing to have Farrow talk with his therapist about whether he had crossed an ethical line. There was no risk of introducing the idea of ethical responsibility.

Movie critics and cultural observers have noted how often in Allen's films older men groom and become sexually involved with young women, often 17 to 18 years old, and how sophisticated people followed Allen's lead in normalizing those relationships (Bellafonte, 2021). Like many others, I loved Woody Allen's films and, although I felt queasy about it, was insensitive to the exploitation in those relationships. Perhaps millions like me would have woken up sooner if Allen's therapists, over decades of treatment, had been more attuned to the ethical dimensions of his life experience—or if the therapist who viewed those nude photographs had broken ranks with therapists of his time and engaged Allen in a conversation about whether it was ethical and healthy to live in a self-created moral universe.

THE CASE OF MONICA LEWINSKY

While Woody Allen's therapy may have had a cultural impact, arguably the most consequential lack of ethical consultation occurred in the case of Monica Lewinsky, whose affair with President Bill Clinton led to his impeachment and arguably influenced the next presidential election, which Al Gore lost by a small number of votes in one state (Pomper, 2001). We know something about Lewinsky's therapy because the Starr Report, which led to Clinton's impeachment, contained an interview with Lewinsky's therapist, a famous psychologist and author of a number of self-help books (Starr, 1998). (Lewinsky had signed a release for the therapist to speak to the Starr Commission.)

As I read the interview summary, I was struck by the therapist's exclusive focus on protecting Lewinsky from job loss and rejection by Clinton, with no mention of the potential harm the relationship could create for Clinton's wife and daughter—and the country. According to the report, the therapist "counseled Lewinsky not to share this information [about the affair] with anyone except another therapist, *inasmuch as Lewinsky was the only one who could be harmed* [emphasis added]" (Starr, 1998, p. 2). According to the report, while the affair was going on, the therapist "counseled Lewinsky would be discovered and recommended that the two doors be locked" (p. 2).

There was at least one opportunity to discuss the effects of the affair on Clinton's family, but the therapist passed on it:

> The President gave Lewinsky a goodbye speech in which he said that Lewinsky was such a wonderful girl, but that he was concerned about his wife and daughter. [The therapist] believes that the speech was manufactured by the President and not sincere. Lewinsky accepted the speech as true. (Starr, 1998, p. 4)

Although the therapist was circumspect during the Starr Commission interview, she was more expansive in a prior interview with a journalist about her understanding of why Lewinsky engaged in a sexual relationship (that did not include intercourse) with Clinton and how she would have felt and perhaps acted:

> What intern in what country wouldn't [find it irresistible] if the top guy said, "You're adorable, you're wonderful"? It's so seductive, it's so delicious to have a Big Daddy look at you. And then the thing develops. At first you think maybe he just wants to talk to you or something. It develops. . . . I think he [President Clinton] is cute. . . . But if he and I did it, we'd have to have penetration. I'd insist. (Carlson, 1998, para. 2)

I recognize that this is a stunning quote. Assuming that it's accurate, I will refrain from speculating on what was going on for the therapist and just note that it sounds like the authentic/liberated self of the 1960s (see my discussion of this in Chapter 1 of this volume) and that we are far afield here from the relational self and ethical consultation.

I want to be clear that Clinton is morally responsible for using his position of power to invite a 21-year-old intern into a secret extramarital affair. Having said that, what if Lewinsky's therapist had offered her ethical consultation about the current and future harm that this affair would create, not only for her but also for all of those affected, including a country which would be shaken by its disclosure and the subsequent lies and impeachment? Would Lewinsky have avoided the affair or ended it before she started confiding in others who eventually went to investigators? As mentioned, a case can be made that media and public reaction influenced the close presidential election of 2000 (Yioutas & Segvic, 2003)—and with that election, subsequent U.S. and world history. How would our nation's leaders have responded to the 9/11 attacks if they had occurred under President Gore? Would the United States have become involved in the Iraq War? Would we have tackled climate change sooner?

There is a permeable membrane between what we do in our offices and what happens in the personal and public lives of our clients. If we focus only on the immediate self-interest of those who hire us, we fail them and the larger world. When we expand our vision to see our clients as relational selves with responsibilities and commitments beyond their self-interest, we contribute to their wholeness, and we help make the world a more humane and just place for all of us.

References

Acocella, J. (1999). *Creating hysteria: Women and multiple personality disorder*. Jossey-Bass.

Adler, A. (1992). *Understanding human nature*. Oneworld. (Original work published 1927)

Aldarondo, E. (Ed.). (2008). *Advancing social justice through clinical practice*. Routledge.

Allen, W. (Director). (1994). *Bullets over Broadway* [Film]. Miramax.

Amato, P. R. (2010). Research on divorce: Continuing trends and new developments. *Journal of Marriage and the Family, 72*(3), 650–666. https://doi.org/10.1111/j.1741-3737.2010.00723.x

American Psychiatric Association. (2013). *Diagnostic and statistical manual of mental disorders* (5th ed.). American Psychiatric Association Publishing.

Anderson, W. T. (2004). *The upstart spring: Esalen and the human potential movement*. IUniverse.

Bass, E., & Davis, L. (1988). *The courage to heal: A guide for women survivors of sexual abuse*. Harper & Row.

Baucom, D. H., Snyder, D. K., & Gordon, K. C. (2011). *Helping couples get past the affair*. Guilford Press.

Bellafonte, G. (2021, March 5). Why my teenage self gave Woody Allen a pass. *The New York Times*. https://www.nytimes.com/2021/03/05/nyregion/woody-allen-manhattan.html?searchResultPosition=6

Bellah, R. N., Madsen, R., Sullivan, W. M., Swidler, A., & Tipton, S. M. (1985). *Habits of the heart: Individualism and commitment in American life*. University of California Press.

Berger, P., & Luckmann, T. (1966). *The social construction of reality*. Doubleday.

Berkowitz, E. D. (2006). *Something happened: A political and cultural overview of the seventies*. Columbia University Press.

Bikel, O. (Writer & Director). (1995). Divided memories. *Frontline*. PBS.

Bok, S. (1979). *Lying: Moral choice in public and private life*. Vintage Books.

Booth, P., & Amato, P. R. (2001). Parents predivorce relations and offspring postdivorce well-being. *Journal of Marriage and the Family, 63*(1), 197–212. https://doi.org/10.1111/j.1741-3737.2001.00197.x

Boszormenyi-Nagy, I., & Krasner, B. R. (1986). *Between give and take: A clinical guide to contextual therapy.* Brunner/Mazel.

Boyte, H. C. (2005). *Everyday politics: Reconnecting citizens and public life.* University of Pennsylvania Press.

Bronfenbrenner, U. (1979). *The ecology of human development.* Harvard University Press.

Buber, M. (1958). *I and thou* (2nd ed.) (R. G. Smith, Trans.). Charles Scribner's Sons.

Campbell, S. (2019). *But it's your family . . .: Cutting ties with toxic family members and loving yourself in the aftermath.* Morgan James.

Carlson, T. (1998, March 23). Monica's therapist speaks. *The Washington Examiner.* https://www.washingtonexaminer.com/tag/tucker-carlson?source=%2Fweekly-standard%2Fmonicas-therapist-speaks

cavettbiter. (2007, October 19). *Dick & Woody on psychoanalysis* [Video]. YouTube. https://www.youtube.com/watch?v=Ss8fYIKlRdo

Chen, S., Boucher, H. C., & Tapias, M. P. (2006). The relational self revealed: Integrative conceptualization and implications for interpersonal life. *Psychological Bulletin, 132*(2), 151–179. https://doi.org/10.1037/0033-2909.132.2.151

Cohen, L. (2008). *A consumers' republic: The politics of mass consumption in postwar America.* Viking.

Comas-Díaz, L. (2020). Liberation psychotherapy. In L. Comas-Díaz & E. Torres Rivera (Eds.), *Liberation psychology: Theory, method, practice, and social justice* (pp. 169–185). American Psychological Association. https://doi.org/10.1037/0000198-010

Conroy, P. (1978, November 1). Anatomy of a divorce. *Atlanta Magazine.* https://www.atlantamagazine.com/great-reads/anatomy-of-a-divorce/

Copen, C. E., Daniels, K., Vespa, J., & Mosher, W. D. (2012). *First marriages in the United States: Data from the 2006–2010 National Survey of Family Growth* (National Health Statistics Reports, No. 49). National Center for Health Statistics. https://www.cdc.gov/nchs/data/nhsr/nhsr049.pdf

Crisp, R. (Ed.). (2015). *The Oxford handbook of the history of ethics.* Oxford University Press.

Davis, S. D., Fife, S. T., Whiting, J. B., & Bradford, K. P. (2021). Way of being and the therapeutic pyramid: Expanding the application of a common factors meta-model. *Journal of Marital and Family Therapy, 47*, 69–84. https://doi.org/10.1111/jmft.12466

DePaulo, B. M. (2018). Lying in social psychology. In J. Meibauer (Ed.), *The Oxford handbook of lying* (pp. 436–445). Oxford University Press.

Dewey, J. (1993). *The political writings.* Hackett.

Dick, K., & Ziering, A. (Directors). (2021). Episode 3 [TV series episode]. In A. Herdy (Producer), *Allen v. Farrow.* HBO.

Doherty, W. J. (1993). I'm O.K., you're O.K., but what about the kids? *The Family Therapy Networker, 17,* 46–53.

Doherty, W. J. (1995). *Soul searching: Why psychotherapy must promote moral responsibility.* Basic Books.

Doherty, W. J. (1999, May/June). Divided loyalties: The challenge of stepfamily life. *Psychotherapy Networker, 54,* 33–38. https://dohertyrelationshipinstitute.com/wp-content/uploads/2019/11/stepfamilies.pdf

Doherty, W. J. (2000). *Take back your kids: Confident parenting in turbulent times.* Sorin Books.

Doherty, W. J. (2002a, November/December). Bad couples therapy: How to avoid doing it. *Psychotherapy Networker,* 26–33. https://dohertyrelationshipinstitute.com/wp-content/uploads/2019/11/Bad_Couples_Therapy.pdf

Doherty, W. J. (2002b). How therapists harm marriages and what we can do about it. *Journal of Couple & Relationship Therapy, 1*(?), 1–17. https://doi.org/10.1300/J398v01n02_01

Doherty, W. J. (2006, March/April). Couples on the brink: Stopping the marriage-go-round. *Psychotherapy Networker, 70,* 30–39. https://dohertyrelationshipinstitute.com/wp-content/uploads/2019/11/Couples_On_the_Brink_Networker.pdf

Doherty, W. J. (2008, November/December). Beyond the consulting room: Therapists as catalysts for social change. *Psychotherapy Networker,* 28–35.

Doherty, W. (2015, July/August). Reflections on the divorce revolution: Assessing our impact. *Psychotherapy Networker, 39,* 19–25, 42–44.

Doherty, W. (2017a, November/December). Is there hope for a divided America? Tales from the Better Angels bus tour. *Psychotherapy Networker, 54,* 23–29. https://www.psychotherapynetworker.org/magazine/article/1123/is-there-hope-for-a-divided-america

Doherty, W. J. (2017b). New opportunities for therapy in the age of Trump. In B. Lee (Ed.), *The dangerous case of Donald Trump* (pp. 209–216). St. Martin's Press.

Doherty, W. (2017c, January/February). Psychotherapy's pilgrimage: Shaping the consciousness of our time. *Psychotherapy Networker, 67,* 19–31. https://www.psychotherapynetworker.org/magazine/article/1070/psychotherapys-pilgrimage

Doherty, W. J. (2020a). The evolution and current status of systemic family therapy: A sociocultural perspective. In R. B. Miller & R. B. Seedall (Eds.), *Handbook of systemic family therapy: Vol. 1. The profession of systemic family therapy* (pp. 33–49). Wiley. https://doi.org/10.1002/9781119438519.ch2

Doherty, W. J. (2020b). My journey as a citizen therapist. *Journal of Humanistic Psychology, 60*(4), 477–487. https://doi.org/10.1177/0022167819899594

Doherty, W. J., & Carlson, B. Z. (2003). Overscheduled kids and underconnected families. In J. de Graaf (Ed.), *Take back your time: Fighting overwork and time famine in families* (pp. 38–45). Berritt Koehler.

Doherty, W. J., & Harris, S. M. (2017). *Helping couples on the brink of divorce: Discernment counseling for troubled relationships*. American Psychological Association. https://doi.org/10.1037/0000029-000

Doherty, W. J., Mendenhall, T. J., & Berge, J. M. (2010). The Families and Democracy and Citizen Health Care Project. *Journal of Marital and Family Therapy, 36*(4), 389–402. https://doi.org/10.1111/j.1752-0606.2009.00142.x

Edin, K., & Nelson, T. J. (2013). *Doing the best I can: Fatherhood in the inner city*. University of California Press. https://doi.org/10.1525/9780520955134

Engel, G. L. (1977, April 8). The need for a new medical model: A challenge for biomedicine. *Science, 196*(4286), 129–136. https://doi.org/10.1126/science.847460

Felthous, A. R. (2006). Warning a potential victim of a person's dangerousness: Clinician's duty or victim's right? *The Journal of the American Academy of Psychiatry and the Law, 34*(3), 338–348.

Finkel, E. J., Bail, C. A., Cikara, M., Ditto, P. H., Iyengar, S., Klar, S., Mason, L., McGrath, M. C., Nyhan, B., Rand, D. G., Skitka, L. J., Tucker, J. A., Van Bavel, J. J., Wang, C. S., & Druckman, J. N. (2020, October 30). Political sectarianism in America. *Science, 370*(6516), 533–536. https://doi.org/10.1126/science.abe1715

Fowers, B. J. (2005). *Virtue in psychology: Pursing excellence in ordinary practices*. American Psychological Association. https://doi.org/10.1037/11219-000

Fowers, B. J., Anderson, A. R., Lefevor, G. T., & Lang, S. (2015). Beyond harms: Exploring the individual and shared goods of psychotherapy. *The Counseling Psychologist, 43*(3), 380–392. https://doi.org/10.1177/0011000014568202

Freud, S. (1961). *The ego and the id*. W W Norton & Co.

Gerstle, G. (2017). *American crucible: Race and class in the twentieth century*. Princeton University Press.

Gibbon, S., Duggan, C., Stoffers, J., Huband, N., Völlm, B. A., Ferriter, M., & Lieb, K. (2010). Psychological interventions for antisocial personality disorder. *Cochrane Database of Systematic Reviews*. https://doi.org/10.1002/14651858.CD007668.pub2

Giluk, T. L., & Postlethwaite, B. E. (2015). Big five personality and academic dishonesty: A meta-analytic review. *Personality and Individual Differences, 72,* 59–67. https://doi.org/10.1016/j.paid.2014.08.027

Gordon, K. C., Khaddouma, K. M., Baucom, D. H., & Snyder, D. K. (2018). Couple therapy and the treatment of affairs. In A. S. Gurman, J. L. Lebow, & D. L. Snyder (Eds.), *Clinical handbook of couple therapy* (5th ed., pp. 606–634). Guilford Press.

Gottman, J., & Gottman, J. (2021). *The Gottman Method*. The Gottman Institute. https://www.gottman.com/about/the-gottman-method/

Graham, J., Haidt, J., Motyl, M., Meindl, P., Iskiwitch, C., & Mooljman, M. (2018). In K. Gray & J. Graham (Eds.), *Atlas of moral psychology* (pp. 211–222). Guilford Press.

Gray, K., & Graham, J. (Eds.). (2018). *Atlas of moral psychology*. Guilford Press.

Haidt, J. (2012). *The righteous mind: Why good people are divided by politics and religion*. Pantheon.

Haidt, J., & Joseph, C. (2007). The moral mind: How five sets of innate intuitions guide the development of many culture-specific virtues, and perhaps even modules. *The Innate Mind, 3*, 367–391.

Haritaworn, C. L., & Klesse, C. (2006). Poly/logue: A critical introduction to polyamory. *Sexualities, 9*(5), 515–529. https://doi.org/10.1177/1363460706069963

Harris, S. M., Crabtree, S. A., Bell, N. K., Allen, S. M., & Roberts, K. M. (2017). Seeking clarity and confidence in the divorce decision making process. *Journal of Divorce & Remarriage, 58*(2), 83–95. https://doi.org/10.1080/10502556.2016.1268015

Hart, C., Jones, J., Terrizzi, J., & Curtis, D. (2019). Development of the Lying in Everyday Situations Scale. *The American Journal of Psychology, 132*(3), 343–352. https://doi.org/10.5406/amerjpsyc.132.3.0343

Hemez, P. (2016). *Attitudes towards marital infidelity*. https://www.bgsu.edu/ncfmr/resources/data/family-profiles/hemez-attitudes-marital-infidelity-fp-16-12.html

Hertlein, K. M., Wetchler, J. L., & Piercy, F. P. (2005). Infidelity. *Journal of Couple & Relationship Therapy, 4*(2–3), 5–16. https://doi.org/10.1300/J398v04n02_02

Hetherington, M., & Weiler, J. (2018). *Prius versus pickup: How answers to four simple questions explain America's great divide*. Houghton Mifflin Harcourt.

Hillman, J., & Ventura, M. (1993). *We've had a hundred years of psychotherapy— And the world's getting worse*. HarperOne.

Janoff-Bulman, R., & Carnes, N. C. (2018). The model of moral motives: A map of the moral domain. In K. Gray & J. Graham (Eds.), *Atlas of moral psychology* (pp. 223–230). Guilford Press.

Johnson, S. (2013). *Love sense: The revolutionary new science of romantic relationships*. Little Brown.

Jones, D. (1966). Freud's theory of moral conscience. *Philosophy, 41*(155), 34–57. https://doi.org/10.1017/S0031819100066134

Kahneman, D. (2017). *Thinking, fast and slow*. Farrar, Straus & Giroux.

Knapp, S. J., VandeCreek, L. D., & Fingerhut, R. (2017). *Practical ethics for psychologists: A positive approach* (3rd ed.). American Psychological Association.

Kohlberg, L. (1984). *Essays in moral development*. Harper & Row.

Lageman, A. G. (1993). *The moral dimensions of marriage and family therapy*. University Press of America.

Lasch, C. (1979). *The culture of narcissism*. Warner Books.

Lee, C. (Ed.). (2018). *Counseling for social justice* (3rd ed.). American Counseling Association Foundation.

Lerner, M. (1991). *Surplus powerlessness: The psychodynamics of everyday life— And the psychology of individual and social transformation*. Humanities Press International.

Levinas, E. (1969). *Totality and infinity: An essay on exteriority* (A. Lingis, Trans.). Duquesne University Press.

London, P. (1964). *The modes and morals of psychotherapy.* Holt, Rinehart & Winston.

London, P. (1986). *The modes and morals of psychotherapy.* Routledge.

Marks, P. (1993, April 20). Psychologist is pressured on views by judge in Allen custody case. *The New York Times*, p. 3.

Mason, L. (2018). *Uncivil agreement: How politics became our identity.* University of Chicago Press. https://doi.org/10.7208/chicago/9780226524689.001.0001

May, R. (1992). Foreward. In D. K. Freedheim (Ed.), *History of psychotherapy: A century of change* (pp. xx–xxvii). American Psychological Association.

McCoy, S. P., & Aamodt, M. G. (2010). A comparison of law enforcement divorce rates with those of other occupations. *Journal of Criminal Psychology, 25*(1), 1–16. https://doi.org/10.1007/s11896-009-9057-8

McDaniel, S. H., Doherty, W. J., & Hepworth, J. (2014). *Medical family therapy and integrated care* (2nd ed.). American Psychological Association.

McGoldrick, M., & Hardy, K. V. (2008). *Re-visioning family therapy: Race, culture, and gender in clinical practice* (2nd ed.). Guilford Press.

Meade, G. H. (1956). *On social psychology: Selected papers* (A. Straus, Ed.). University of Chicago Press.

Mitchell, S. A., & Aron, L. (Eds.). (1999). *Relational psychoanalysis: The emergence of a tradition.* Routledge.

Moller, N. P., & Vossler, A. (2015). Defining infidelity in research and couple counseling: A qualitative study. *Journal of Sex & Marital Therapy, 41*(5), 487–497. https://doi.org/10.1080/0092623X.2014.931314

Murphy, W. W. (2016). *Consumer culture and society.* Sage.

Narvaez, D. (2010). Moral complexity: The fatal attraction of truthiness and the importance of mature moral functioning. *Perspectives on Psychological Science, 5*(2), 163–181. https://doi.org/10.1177/1745691610362351

National Divorce Decision-Making Project. (2015). *What are they thinking? A national survey of married individuals who are thinking about divorce.* Family Studies Center, Brigham Young University. https://brightspotcdn.byu.edu/c4/c1/20255b7a43f19f6045a594dfe755/what-are-they-thinking-final-digital.pdf

Nichols, M. W. (1994). *The mystery of goodness and the positive moral consequences of psychotherapy.* Norton.

Noddings, N. (1984). *Caring: A feminine approach to ethics and moral education.* University of California Press.

Perel, E. (2017). *The state of affairs: Rethinking infidelity.* Harper.

Perls, F. (1969). *Gestalt therapy verbatim.* Real People Press.

Peteet, J. R. (2004). *Doing the right thing: An approach to moral issues in mental health treatment.* American Psychiatric Association.

Pipher, M. (2008). *The shelter of each other.* Riverhead Books.

Pomper, G. J. (2001). The 2000 presidential election: Why Gore lost. *Political Science Quarterly, 116*(2), 201–223. https://doi.org/10.2307/798059

Putnam, R. D. (2001). *Bowling alone: The collapse and revival of American community.* Simon & Schuster.

Putnam, R. D. (2016). *Our kids: The American dream in crisis.* Vintage.

Putnam, R. D. (2020). *The upswing: How America came together a century ago and how we can do it again.* Simon & Schuster.

Richardson, F. C., Fowers, B. J., & Guignon, C. B. (1999). *Re-envisioning psychology: Moral dimensions of theory and practice.* Jossey-Bass.

Rieff, P. (1961). *Freud: The mind of the moralist.* Anchor Books.

Rieff, P. (1966). *The triumph of the therapeutic: Uses of faith after Freud.* Harper & Row.

Rogers, C. (1961). *Client-centered therapy.* Houghton Mifflin.

Rogers, C. (1990). A client centered/person centered approach to therapy. In H. Kirschenbaum & V. L. Henderson (Eds.), *The Carl Rogers reader* (pp. 135–152). Houghton Mifflin.

Safer, J. (2019). *I love you, but I hate your politics.* Biteback Publishing.

Schwartz, R. S. (2005). Psychotherapy and social support: Unsettling questions. *Harvard Review of Psychiatry, 13*(5), 272–279. https://doi.org/10.1080/10673220500326458

Serota, K. B., & Levine, T. R. (2015). A few prolific liars: Variation in the prevalence of lying. *Language and Social Psychology, 34*(2), 138–157. https://doi.org/10.1177/0261927X14528804

Shackelford, T. K., LeBlanc, G. J., & Drass, E. (2000). Emotional reactions to infidelity. *Cognition and Emotion, 14*(5), 643–659. https://doi.org/10.1080/02699930050117657

Sheehy, G. (1976). *Passages: Predictable crisis of adult life.* Bantam Books.

Siegel, D. J. (2015). *The developing mind: How relationships and the brain interact to shape who we are* (2nd ed.). Guilford Press.

Slife, B. D., & Wiggins, B. J. (2009). Taking relationship seriously in psychotherapy: Radical relationality. *Journal of Contemporary Psychotherapy, 39*(1), 17–24. https://doi.org/10.1007/s10879-008-9100-6

Spring, J. A. (2013). *After the affair* (2nd ed.). Harper Paperbacks.

Stanley, S. M. (2005). *The power of commitment.* Jossey-Bass.

Starr, K. (1998). *The Starr report: The official report of the Independent Counsel's investigation of the President.* Prima Pub. https://www.govinfo.gov/content/pkg/GPO-CDOC-105hdoc316/pdf/GPO-CDOC-105hdoc316-12.pdf

Steele, H., & Steele, M. (2018). *Handbook of attachment-based interventions.* Guilford Press.

Steigerwald, D. (1995). *The sixties and the end of modern America.* St. Martin's Press.

Suhler, C. L., & Churchland, P. (2011). Can innate, modular "foundations" explain morality? Challenges for Haidt's moral foundations theory. *Journal of Cognitive Neuroscience, 23*(9), 2103–2116. https://doi.org/10.1162/jocn.2011.21637

Taylor, C. (1992). *The ethics of authenticity*. Harvard University Press.

Timm, T., & Blow, A. (1999). Self-of-the-therapist work: A balance between removing restraints and identifying resources. *Contemporary Family Therapy, 21*(3), 331–351. https://doi.org/10.1023/A:1021960315503

Tran, P., Judge, M., & Kashima, Y. (2019). Commitment in relationships: An updated meta-analysis of the investment model. *Personal Relationships, 26*(1), 158–180. https://doi.org/10.1111/pere.12268

Vaughn, D. (1990). *Uncoupling*. Vintage.

Wall, J., Needham, T., Browning, D. S., & James, S. (1999). The ethics of relationality: The moral views of therapists engaged in marital and family therapy. *Family Relations, 48*(2), 139–149. https://doi.org/10.2307/585077

Wallach, M. A., & Wallach, L. (1983). *Psychology's sanction for selfishness: The error of egoism in theory and therapy*. W. H. Freeman.

Weiner-Davis, M. (2002). *The divorce remedy*. Simon & Schuster.

Wilcoxon, A., Remley, T. P., & Gladding, S. T. (2011). *Ethical, legal, and professional issues in the practice of marriage and family therapy* (5th ed.). Pearson.

Wilson, J. Q. (1993). *The moral sense*. Free Press. https://doi.org/10.2307/2938952

Witters, D. (2017). *Americans' well-being declines in 2017*. Gallup. https://news.gallup.com/poll/221588/americans-declines-2017.aspx

Wolfe, A. (1989). *Whose keeper? Social science and moral obligation*. University of California Press.

Wright, L. (1994). *Remembering Satan*. Knopf.

Wu, T. (2017). *The attention merchants: The epic scramble to get inside our heads*. Vintage.

Wylie, M. S. (1993, September/October). The shadow of a doubt. *The Family Therapy Networker, 17*(18–29), 70–73.

Yioutas, J., & Segvic, I. (2003). Revisiting the Clinton/Lewinsky scandal: The convergence of agenda setting and framing. *Journalism & Mass Communication Quarterly, 80*(3), 567–582. https://doi.org/10.1177/107769900308000306

Zaretsky, E. (2005). *Secrets of the soul: A social and cultural history of psychoanalysis*. Vintage.

Index

About the Author

William J. Doherty, PhD, is a professor in the Department of Family Social Science and director of the Citizen Professional Center at the University of Minnesota. He is a practicing psychologist and marriage and family therapist and is cofounder of The Doherty Relationship Institute and the nonprofit Braver Angels. He has made many appearances in media outlets and has written 15 other books, including *Helping Couples on the Brink of Divorce: Discernment Counseling for Troubled Relationships* (2017). Dr. Doherty is past president of the National Council on Family Relations and the recipient of the Lifetime Achievement Award from the American Family Therapy Academy. Visit his website (https://dohertyrelationshipinstitute.com/).